Neonatal Anthropometry for the Chinese

T. F. Fok

MBBS, MD, FRCP(Edin), FRCP(Lond), FRCPCH, FHKCPaed, FHKAM(Paed)

P. C. Ng

MB ChB, MD(Leeds, UK), FRCP(Edin), FRCP(Lond), FRCPCH, FHKCPaed, FHKAM(Paed)

K. L. E. Hon

MBBS, FAAP, PGDipAvMed(Otago), DABPed(Ped Crit Care Med), FHKC Paed, FHKAM(Paed)

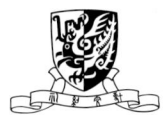

The Chinese University Press

Neonatal Anthropometry for the Chinese
By T. F. Fok, P. C. Ng and K. L. E. Hon

© **The Chinese University of Hong Kong,** 2007

ISBN 978–962–996–335–4

THE CHINESE UNIVERSITY PRESS
The Chinese University of Hong Kong
SHA TIN, N.T., HONG KONG
Fax: +852 2603 6692
　　　+852 2603 7355
E-mail: cup@cuhk.edu.hk
Web-site: www.chineseupress.com

Printed in Hong Kong

CONTENTS

PREFACE

Anthropometric measurements of growth parameters form an integral and vital part of paediatric practice and research. It is important to know the norms of vital parameters in order to appreciate abnormalities when they arise. Knowledge of these data relevant to the local population is especially essential because the application of different ethnic norms to local population may often lead to erroneous observations and decisions.

This book serves the exact role of improvising a comprehensive and up-to-date reference for our local paediatricians and health care professionals. The data are extracted from a number of our published articles, collected by an admirable joint effort of the neonatal services of many local hospitals.

It is hoped that health care professionals will find this book useful and indispensable for their day-to-day practices in the care of sick and healthy neonates alike.

We would like to express our thanks to the Health Care Promotion Fund Committee, Hospital Authority for their supports, the Hong Kong Neonatal Measurements Working Group for their hard work, and Mr Eric Wong of the Centre of Clinical Trials and Epidemiological Research for his important contributions to the construction of all the percentile curves.

T. F. Fok
P. C. Ng
K. L. E. Hon

LIST OF PARTICIPATING HOSPITALS

- Caritas Medical Centre
- Hong Kong Sanatorium
- Kwong Wah Hospital
- Pamela Youde Nethersole Eastern Hospital
- Prince of Wales Hospital
- Princess Margaret Hospital
- Queen Elizabeth Hospital
- Queen Mary Hospital
- Tsan Yuk Hospital
- Tuen Mun Hospital
- Union Hospital
- United Christian Hospital

Members of the Hong Kong Neonatal Measurements Working Group

Chan AKH (Caritas Medical Centre), Tsao YC (Hong Kong Sanatorium), Yuen RKN (Kwong Wah Hospital), Tong CT (Our Lady of Maryknoll Hospital), Young BWY, Ho HT (Pamela Youde Nethersole Eastern Hospital), Fok TF, Ng PC, Hon KLE, Chang AMY (Prince of Wales Hospital), Chow CB (Princess Margaret Hospital), Lee WH (Queen Elizabeth Hospital), Lam BCC (Queen Mary Hospital and Tsan Yuk Hospital), Kwong NS (Tuen Mun Hospital), Lee AKY (Union Hospital), Chan HB (United Christian Hospital)

ACKNOWLEDGEMENTS

The study was supported by a grant from the Health Care and Promotion Fund Committee, the Hospital Authority, Hong Kong. The printing of the *Neonatal Anthropometry for the Chinese* was sponsored by Mead Johnson Nutritionals Representative Office, Hong Kong.

INTRODUCTION

Growth is defined as an increase in size over time. Size at birth reflects two factors: gestational length and fetal growth. The evaluation of the somatic growth of newborns requires a standard of neonatal size in relation to gestational age. The growth of different parts of the body during intra-uterine life follows a predictable schedule, and most syndromes with dysmorphic features have recognizable patterns of disturbed and disproportionate growth and development at birth.

The aim of this book is to provide a serial gestational age-specific standard of physical measurements for local Chinese newborns. These measurements include birth weight, head circumference, body length and other physical measurements with clinical application including those reflecting the skeletal growth of the face, trunk and limbs, and for males, the penile length. These physical parameters provide useful references and aid dysmorphology diagnosis in newborns of ethnic Chinese origin.

SUBJECTS AND METHODS

The study was approved by the Ethics Committee on Clinical Research, The Chinese University of Hong Kong, and the Ethics Committee of the participating hospitals. In Hong Kong, all child births take place in the maternity units of 20 hospitals. During the study period, about 70% of the newborns were born in the 10 public hospitals; the remaining 30% were born in the 10 private hospitals. To ensure that the sample selected truly represented the newborn population in Hong Kong, the babies were recruited from the maternity units of all 10 public hospitals and 2 randomly selected private hospitals.

All the measurements were carried out by 2 teams of field workers according to the method described by Hall et al. (Hall JG 1989), each consisting of 2 investigators who had received training in the use of all measuring equipment. The precision of their measurements was assessed by establishing the inter-observer agreement of the measurements obtained from the first 100 infants. In random sequence, the teams were stationed in each of the participating public hospitals for 2 months and attempts were made to capture all eligible infants born during that period. Thus, the study would capture about one-sixth of the annual deliveries in each of the hospitals. The antenatal history and the condition of each infant were carefully evaluated. A data sheet was used to document the maternal and paternal demographic data as well as the medical and pregnancy history of the mothers. In order to obtain a reasonable sample of infants born in the private hospitals, measurement in the 2 participating private hospitals lasted for 1 year. Logistically it was not possible to include more private hospitals, where the newborn infants were under the care of a large number of private obstetricians and paediatricians.

The main study lasted for 2 years from October 1998 to September 2000. At the end of 2 years, it was realized that the number of infants <35 weeks of gestation was relatively small. The study was then extended for 9 more months until June 2001 to enroll more preterm infants.

Singleton newborns of ethnic Chinese origin with gestation 24–43 weeks were eligible for the study provided informed consent was given by the parents. Infants with the following conditions were excluded: [1] moribund condition at birth, [2] major congenital malformations, [3] chromosomal abnormalities, and [4] gestational age impossible to determine. Infants born to mothers with medical conditions or complications of pregnancy were not excluded since the aim of the study was to construct community-at-large percentile charts rather than those of a "healthy" population.

ASSESSMENT OF GESTATIONAL AGE

Gestational age was calculated as completed weeks, and estimated from the findings of early dating ultrasound performed before 20 weeks of gestation when available. When this was not available, gestational age was calculated from the maternal last menstrual date if the mother had regular menstrual cycles and was certain of her menstrual history. The gestation of each infant was also assessed postnatally using the new Ballard score, which had been evaluated in our Neonatal Unit and found to be applicable for Chinese infants. Only infants whose calculated gestation agreed within 2 weeks with that assessed postnatally were included.

STATISTICS

The LMS method using maximum penalized likelihood was used to perform model fitting of the anthropometric centiles for the physical parameters. The LMS method estimates the measurement centiles in terms of 3 age-sex-specific cubic spline curves: the *L* curve (Box-Cox power to transform the data that follow a normal distribution), *M* curve (median) and *S* curve (coefficient of variation). In brief, if *Y(t)* denotes an independent positive data (e.g. birth weight) at *t* gestation weeks, the distribution of *Y(t)* can be summarized by a normally distributed SD score (*Z*) as follows:

$$Z = \frac{[Y(t) \, / \, M(t)]L(t) - 1}{L(t)S(t)}$$

Once the *L(t), M(t), and S(t)* have been estimated for each gestation *t*, the 100αth centile at *t* gestation weeks could be derived from

$$C_{100\alpha}(t) = M(t)[1 + L(t)S(t)Z_{\alpha}]^{1/L(t)}$$

where Z_{α} is the α centile of the normal distribution (for example for the 97th centile, $\alpha=0.75$ and $Z_{\alpha}=1.88$).

BIRTH WEIGHT,
HEAD CIRCUMFERENCE
&
BODY LENGTH

BIRTH WEIGHT

Definition	Weight or heaviness at birth measured in grams.
Instrument	Electronic weighing scale.
Remark	Babies were weighed naked immediately after birth using an electronic weighing scale accurate to 5 g, which was checked and calibrated regularly.

Birth weight (g)

	Boys			Girls		
Gestation (wk)	N	Mean	SD	N	Mean	SD
24	9	664	87	12	734	44
25	16	775	87	16	786	146
26	12	886	64	11	803	101
27	19	1109	184	18	935	174
28	27	1156	168	19	116	170
29	26	1303	200	36	1227	154
30	51	1476	190	24	1460	282
31	41	1640	261	25	1478	266
32	36	1896	399	45	1711	364
33	89	2057	374	65	1975	302
34	101	2234	354	110	2213	362
35	148	2514	415	133	2423	455
36	275	2803	419	211	2735	395
37	432	3053	413	351	2929	389
38	1054	3204	402	872	3071	357
39	1304	3291	383	1218	3198	365
40	1179	3415	400	1098	3278	388
41	544	3518	429	505	3342	386
42	115	3520	416	92	3423	415

Fok TF, So HK, Wong E, Ng PC, Chang A, Lau J, Chow CB, Lee WH; Hong Kong Neonatal Measurements Working Group. Updated gestational age specific birth weight, crown-heel length, and head circumference of Chinese newborns. Arch Dis Child Fetal Neonatal Ed 2003;88:F229–36.

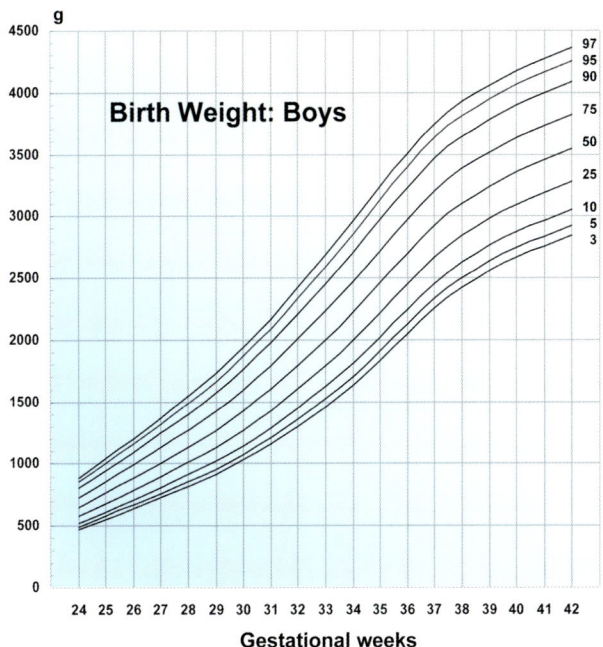

Birth Weight: Boys

Gestational weeks

Birth Weight: Girls

Gestational weeks

BODY LENGTH (CROWN-HEEL LENGTH)

Definition	Length of supine body measured in millimetres.
Instrument	Neonatometer.
Remark	The distance from the top of the head to the sole of the foot with the baby lying on the back with hips and knees extended.
Position	Babies are placed in supine position. One investigator holds the head of the baby, while the other straightens the legs of the baby with one hand, and moves the footblock towards the heel of the babies with the other hand. Heads are held in the Frankfurt horizontal position, (i.e. the lower edge of the bony orbit and the ear are in the same vertical plane).

Body length (mm)

Gestation (wk)	Boys			Girls		
	N	Mean	SD	N	Mean	SD
24	9	322	31	12	333	9
25	16	345	18	16	354	11
26	12	352	13	11	355	13
27	19	373	14	18	358	17
28	27	378	20	19	376	22
29	26	403	25	36	382	19
30	51	408	18	24	405	11
31	41	427	22	25	410	21
32	36	434	28	45	425	21
33	89	447	27	65	444	19
34	101	455	21	110	455	23
35	148	472	21	133	466	24
36	275	482	20	211	481	19
37	432	493	19	351	485	19
38	1054	500	17	872	491	17
39	1304	505	17	1218	498	17
40	1179	511	17	1098	502	16
41	544	514	17	505	504	15
42	115	516	18	92	508	16

Fok TF, So HK, Wong E, Ng PC, Chang A, Lau J, Chow CB, Lee WH; Hong Kong Neonatal Measurements Working Group. Updated gestational age specific birth weight, crown-heel length, and head circumference of Chinese newborns. Arch Dis Child Fetal Neonatal Ed 2003;88:F229–36.

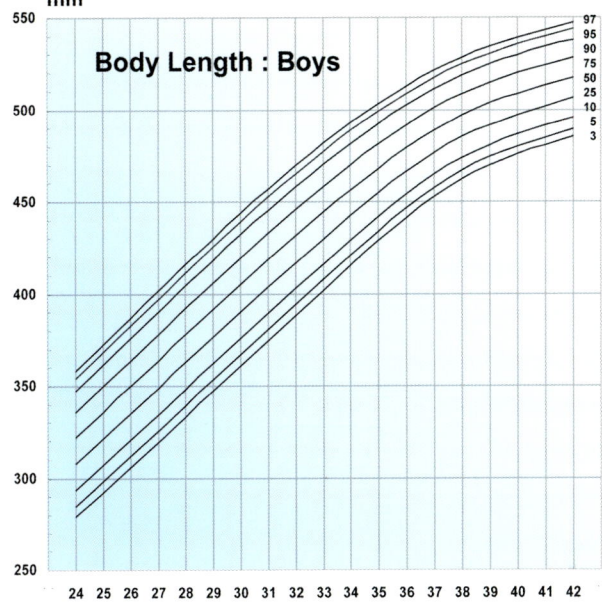

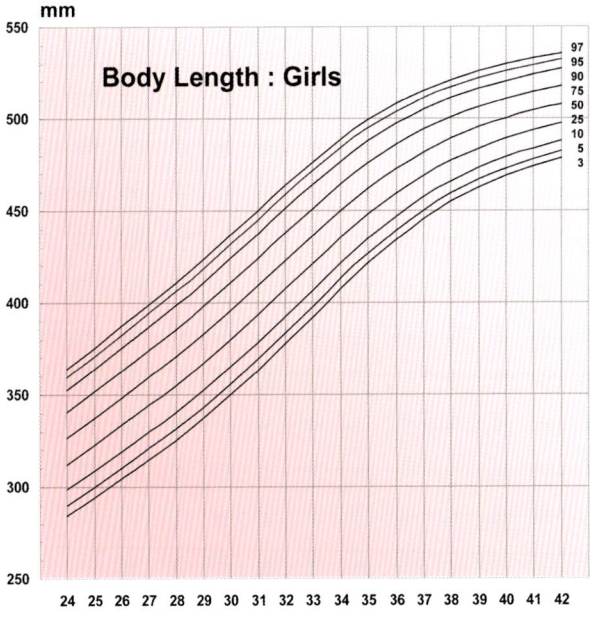

HEAD CIRCUMFERENCE (OCCIPITOFRONTAL CIRCUMFERENCE)

Definition	Maximum circumference of the head measured in millimetres.
Instrument	Inelastic tape measure.
Remark	The maximum head circumference (usually horizontal just above the eyebrow ridges) is measured from just above the glabella area to the area near the top of the occipital bone (opisthocranion), recorded to the nearest millimetre.
Position	Babies are measured lying supine.

Head circumference (mm)

	Boys			Girls		
Gestation (wk)	N	Mean	SD	N	Mean	SD
24	9	226	5	12	234	17
25	16	237	8	16	241	16
26	12	248	10	11	238	8
27	19	253	15	18	250	8
28	27	262	14	19	257	12
29	26	271	16	36	268	13
30	51	281	14	24	281	16
31	41	290	15	25	284	20
32	36	300	20	45	293	14
33	89	307	16	65	304	13
34	101	312	13	110	311	13
35	148	321	15	133	321	14
36	275	331	14	211	328	11
37	432	336	11	351	332	11
38	1054	341	12	872	335	11
39	1304	343	11	1218	338	11
40	1179	347	12	1098	340	11
41	544	350	12	505	343	11
42	115	349	12	92	345	13

Fok TF, So HK, Wong E, Ng PC, Chang A, Lau J, Chow CB, Lee WH; Hong Kong Neonatal Measurements Working Group. Updated gestational age specific birth weight, crown-heel length, and head circumference of Chinese newborns. Arch Dis Child Fetal Neonatal Ed 2003;88:F229–36.

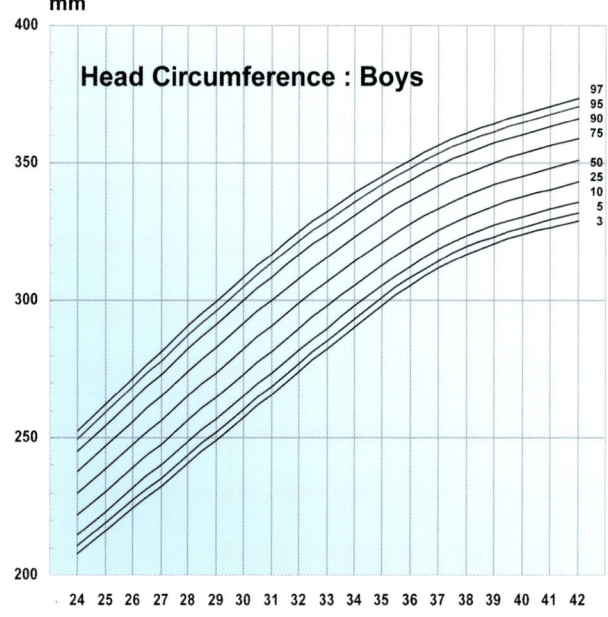

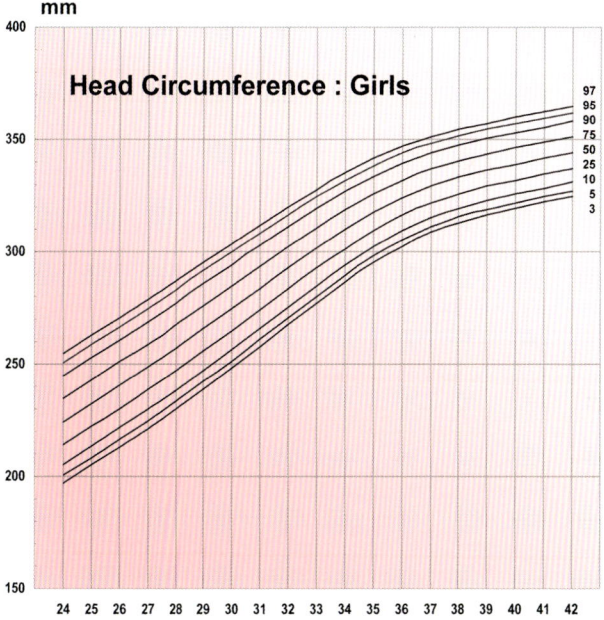

TRUNK

- Chest Circumference
- Inner-nipple Distance
- Sternal Length
- Abdominal Circumference

CHEST CIRCUMFERENCE

Definition	Circumference of chest measured in millimetres.
Instrument	Inelastic tape measure.
Remark	The circumference around the upper body at the level of the nipples and below the inferior angle of the scapula during quiet respiration.
Position	Babies are measured lying supine on a flat surface, in mid-expiration.

Chest circumference (mm)

Gestation (wk)	Boys			Girls		
	N	Mean	SD	N	Mean	SD
26	12	213	8	11	214	7
27	19	223	5	18	220	20
28	27	233	24	19	228	12
29	26	243	12	36	236	15
30	51	252	11	24	244	23
31	41	262	22	25	254	20
32	36	272	21	45	264	24
33	89	281	24	65	275	11
34	101	290	15	110	286	19
35	148	299	22	133	296	23
36	275	307	19	211	305	15
37	432	314	17	351	312	18
38	1054	320	16	872	318	15
39	1304	325	15	1218	323	15
40	1179	330	16	1098	327	15
41	544	334	17	505	330	15
42	115	338	15	92	333	15

Fok TF, Hon KL, Wong E, Ng PC, So HK, Lau J, Chow CB, Lee WH; Hong Kong Neonatal Measurements Working Group. Trunk anthropometry of Hong Kong Chinese infants. Early Hum Dev 2005;81:781–90.

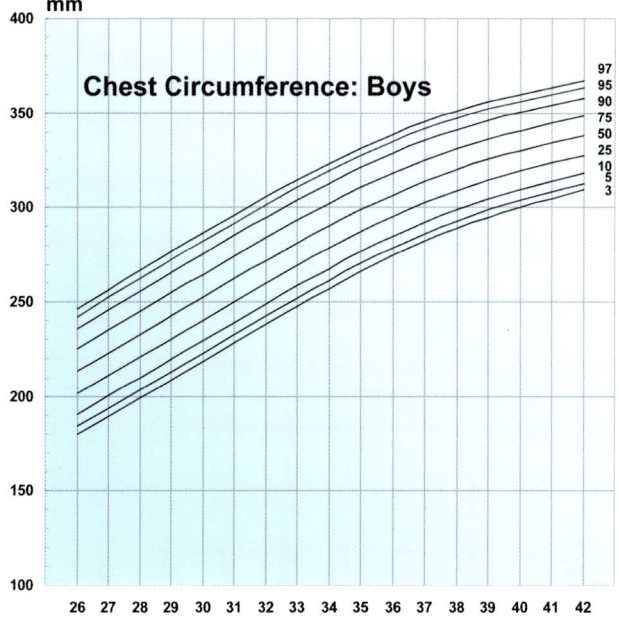

Gestational weeks

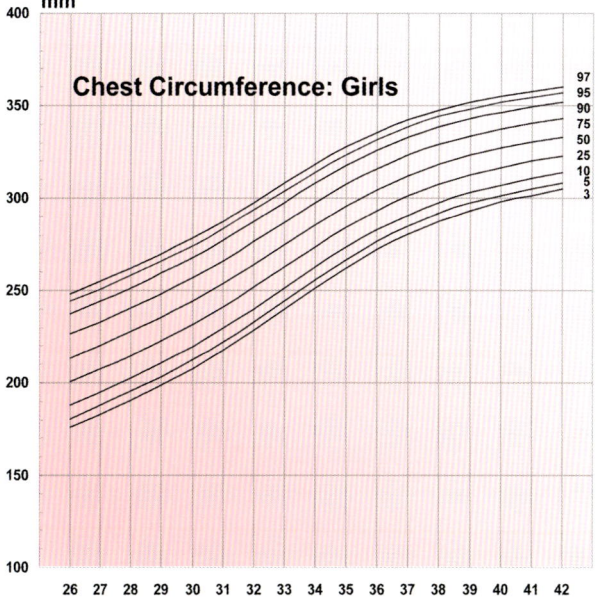

Gestational weeks

11

INTER-NIPPLE DISTANCE

Definition	Distance between the centres of both nipples measured in millimetres.
Instrument	Inelastic tape measure.
Remark	The distance between the centres of the nipples during quiet respiration.
Position	Babies are measured lying supine, in mid-expiration.

Inter-nipple distance (mm)

Gestation (wk)	Boys			Girls		
	N	Mean	SD	N	Mean	SD
26	12	50	4	11	51	4
27	19	53	6	18	53	8
28	27	56	10	19	55	6
29	26	58	4	36	57	5
30	51	61	4	24	59	7
31	41	64	6	25	61	8
32	36	67	6	45	64	7
33	89	69	7	65	67	5
34	101	72	6	110	70	7
35	148	74	6	133	73	8
36	275	76	5	211	75	6
37	432	78	7	351	77	6
38	1054	80	6	872	79	6
39	1304	81	6	1218	80	6
40	1179	83	6	1098	81	6
41	544	84	6	505	82	6
42	115	85	6	92	83	6

Fok TF, Hon KL, Wong E, Ng PC, So HK, Lau J, Chow CB, Lee WH; Hong Kong Neonatal Measurements Working Group. Trunk anthropometry of Hong Kong Chinese infants. Early Hum Dev. 2005;81:781–90.

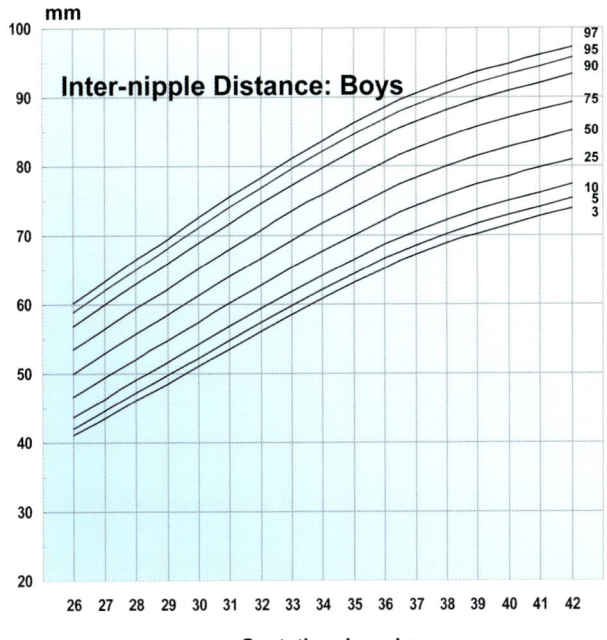

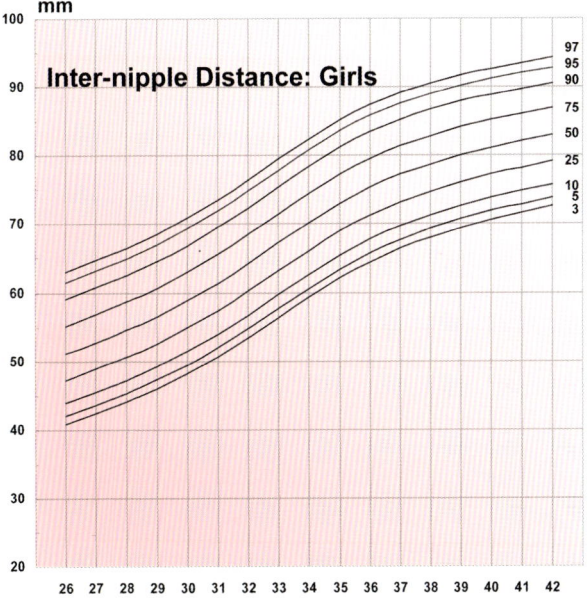

13

STERNAL LENGTH

Definition   Length of the sternum measured in millimetres.
Instrument   Inelastic tape measure.
Remark   The distance from the top of the manubrium to the xiphoid process
               with the baby supine.

Sternal length (mm)							
	Boys				Girls		
Gestation (wk)	N	Mean	SD		N	Mean	SD
26	12	52	2		11	51	11
27	19	54	8		18	53	10
28	27	57	9		19	56	5
29	26	59	4		36	58	8
30	51	62	6		24	61	8
31	41	64	11		25	63	4
32	36	67	6		45	66	9
33	89	69	9		65	68	8
34	101	71	9		110	70	8
35	148	73	7		133	72	7
36	275	75	6		211	74	6
37	432	77	7		351	75	6
38	1054	79	6		872	77	6
39	1304	80	6		1218	78	6
40	1179	82	6		1098	79	6
41	544	83	6		505	80	5
42	115	84	7		92	81	7

Fok TF, Hon KL, Wong E, Ng PC, So HK, Lau J, Chow CB, Lee WH; Hong Kong Neonatal Measurements Working Group. Trunk anthropometry of Hong Kong Chinese infants. Early Hum Dev 2005;81:781–90.

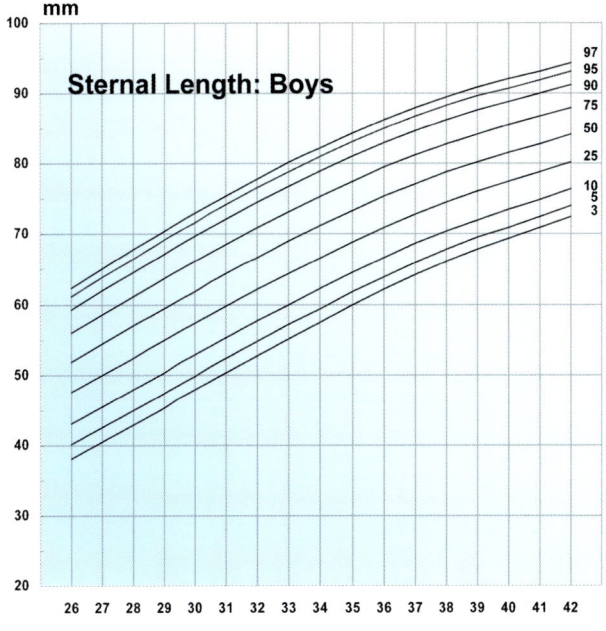

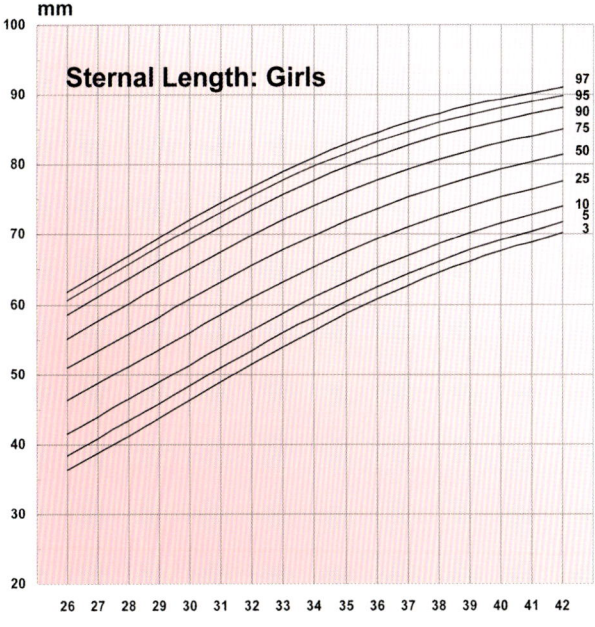

15

ABDOMINAL CIRCUMFERENCE

Definition	Circumference of abdomen measured in millimetres.
Instrument	Inelastic tape measure.
Remark	The circumference around the abdomen at the mid-point between the xiphoid and umbilical cord during quiet respiration.
Position	Babies are measured lying supine, in mid-expiration. No measurement was recorded within half an hour after feeding.

Abdominal circumference (mm)

	Boys			Girls		
Gestation	N	Mean	SD	N	Mean	SD
26	12	207	19	11	211	1
27	19	216	10	18	219	25
28	27	226	8	19	227	18
29	26	237	11	36	236	16
30	51	247	12	24	246	12
31	41	258	18	25	256	22
32	36	269	28	45	267	22
33	89	279	26	65	278	11
34	101	289	18	110	288	20
35	148	297	20	133	297	22
36	275	305	16	211	305	17
37	432	312	17	351	312	18
38	1054	318	17	872	317	16
39	1304	322	16	1218	320	17
40	1179	326	19	1098	323	18
41	544	329	18	505	325	18
42	115	332	18	92	327	18

Fok TF, Hon KL, Wong E, Ng PC, So HK, Lau J, Chow CB, Lee WH; Hong Kong Neonatal Measurements Working Group. Trunk anthropometry of Hong Kong Chinese infants. Early Hum Dev 2005;81:781–90.

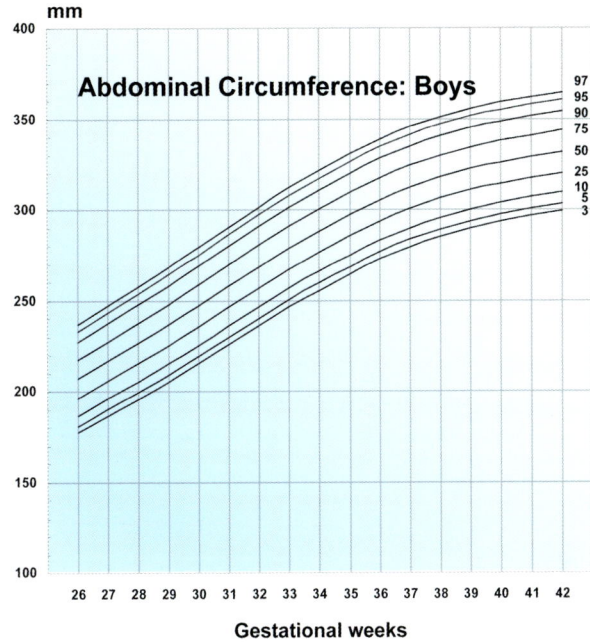

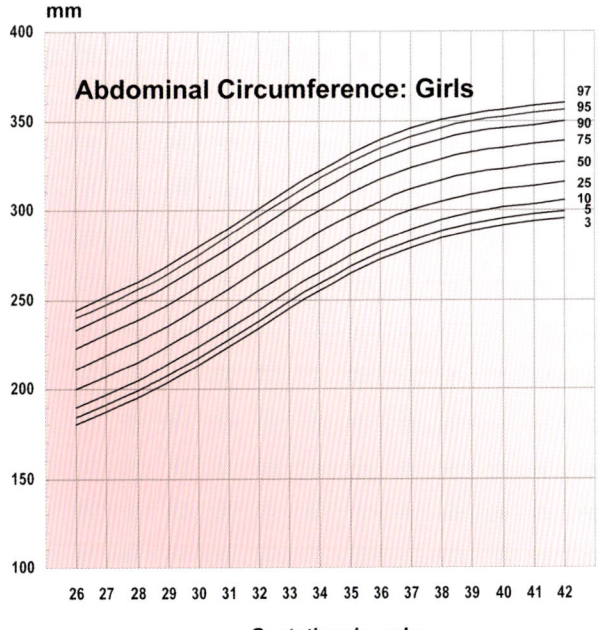

Gestational weeks

17

CRANIOFACIES

- Facial Width, Facial Height
- Outer Canthal Distance
- Inner Canthal Distance
- Palpebral Fissure Length
- Nasal Length, Nasal Width
- Ear Length, Ear Width
- Philtrum Length

All the craniofacial measurements were carried out with the baby's head in the Frankfurt horizontal position. The Frankfurt horizontal position is established when the head is held erect, with the eyes looking forward, so that the lowest margin of the lower bony orbit and the upper margin of the external auditory meatus are in the same horizontal plane.

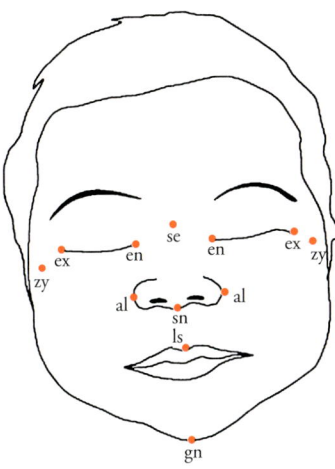

Figure 1

Zygion (zy) is the most lateral point of each zygomatic arch.

Gnathion (gn) is the lowest median landmark on the lower border of the mandible.

Endocanthion (en) is the point at the inner commissure of the eye fissure.

Exocanthion (ex) is the point at the outer commissure of the eye fissure.

Sellion (se) is the deepest landmark located on the bottom of the nasofrontal angle.

Subnasale (sn) is the base of the nose.

Ala (al) is the most lateral point of the ala.

Labiale superius (ls) is the mid-point of the upper vermilion line.

FACIAL WIDTH (BIZYGOMATIC DISTANCE)

Definition   The maximal distance between the most lateral points on the zygomatic arches (zygion) (zy-zy) in millimetres.

Instrument   Spreading caliper.

Remark   The distance between the most lateral points of the zygomatic arches.

Facial width (mm)

Gestation	Boys			Girls		
	N	Mean	SD	N	Mean	SD
33	10	70	5	5	69	3
34	9	72	3	11	72	6
35	16	75	5	15	74	4
36	37	77	5	28	76	4
37	125	79	5	112	78	4
38	241	80	5	234	79	4
39	358	81	5	279	80	4
40	294	81	5	268	80	5
41	138	82	5	120	81	5
42	40	82	4	37	81	4

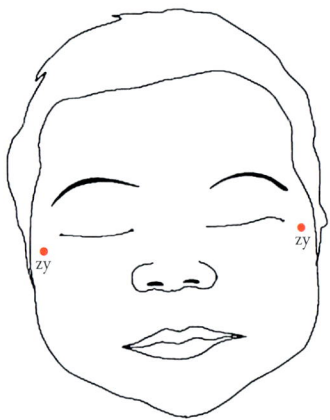

Figure 2

Fok TF, Hon KL, So HK, Wong E, Ng PC, Lee AK, Chang A. Facial anthropometry of Hong Kong Chinese babies. Orthod Craniofac Res 2003;6:164–72.

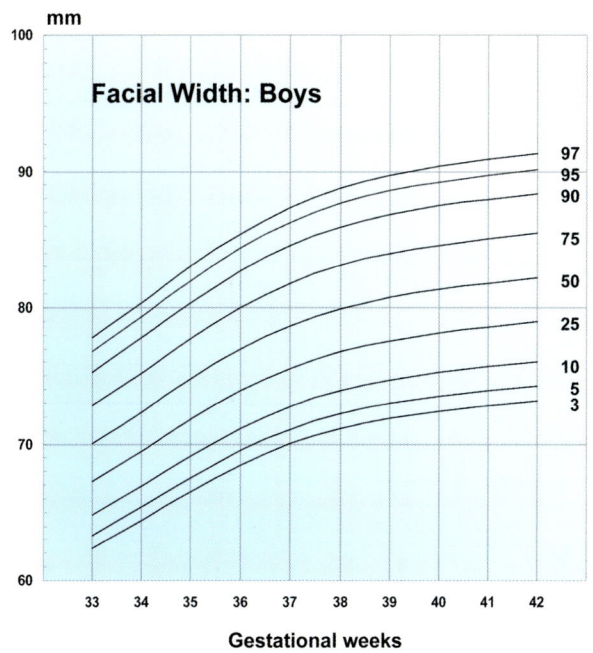

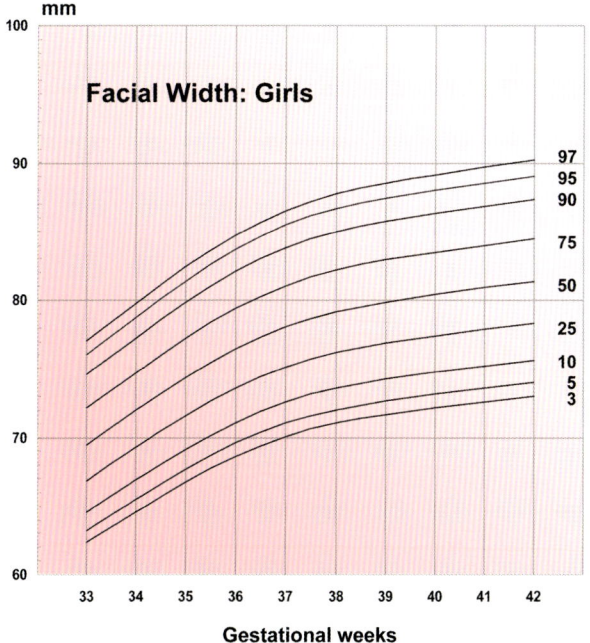

FACIAL HEIGHT

Definition   Distance from the root of the nose (nasion) to the lowest median landmark on the lower border of the mandible (menton or gnathion). Lower two-thirds of craniofacies (se-gn) in millimetres.

Instrument   Spreading caliper.

Remark   The distance from the root of the nose to the inferior border of the mandible in a vertical plane.

Facial height (mm)

Gestation (wk)	Boys			Girls		
	N	Mean	SD	N	Mean	SD
33	10	43	3	5	43	1
34	9	44	3	11	43	2
35	16	44	3	15	44	3
36	37	45	3	28	45	4
37	125	46	4	112	45	3
38	241	46	4	234	46	3
39	358	47	4	279	46	3
40	294	47	4	268	47	4
41	138	47	3	120	47	4
42	40	47	4	37	47	3

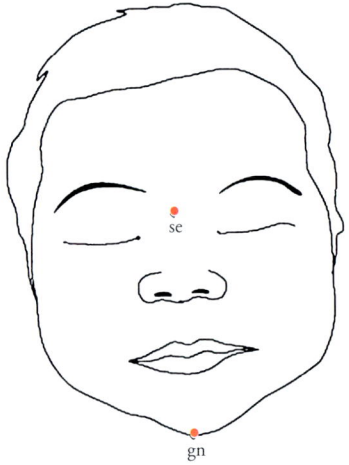

Figure 3

Fok TF, Hon KL, So HK, Wong E, Ng PC, Lee AK, Chang A. *Facial anthropometry of Hong Kong Chinese babies. Orthod Craniofac Res 2003;6:164–72.*

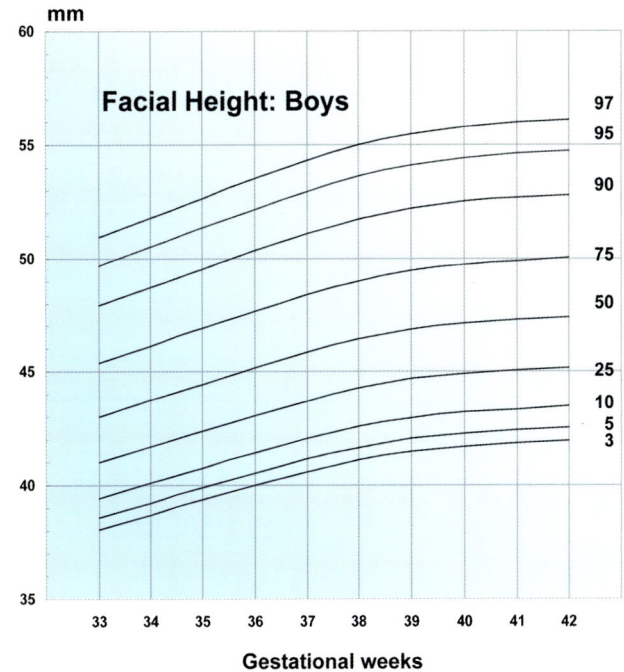

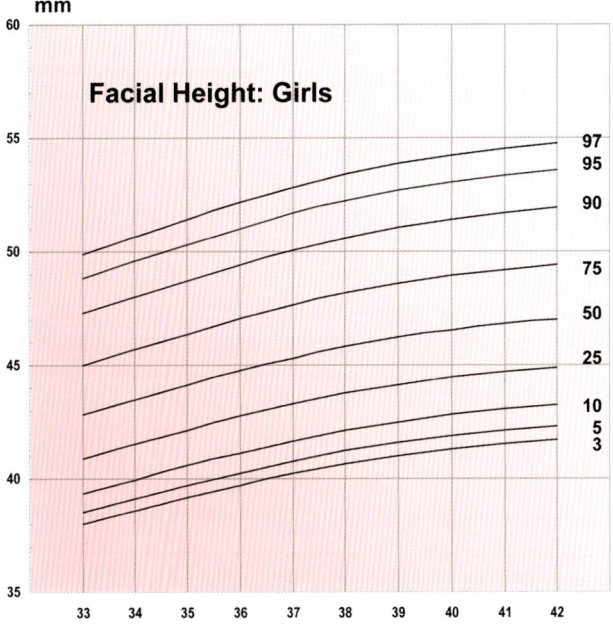

OUTER CANTHAL DISTANCE

Definition   The distance between the outer canthi of the two eyes (ex-ex) in millimetres.

Instrument   Spreading caliper.

Remark   The distance from the most lateral corner of one eye to the most lateral corner of the other eye, in a straight line avoiding the curvature of the face.

Outer canthal distance (mm)

Gestation (wk)	Boys			Girls		
	N	Mean	SD	N	Mean	SD
33	10	58	2	5	56	4
34	9	60	6	11	58	4
35	16	61	3	15	60	4
36	37	62	4	28	62	5
37	125	64	4	112	63	4
38	241	65	4	234	64	4
39	358	66	4	279	65	4
40	294	66	4	268	65	4
41	138	67	4	120	66	4
42	40	67	4	37	66	4

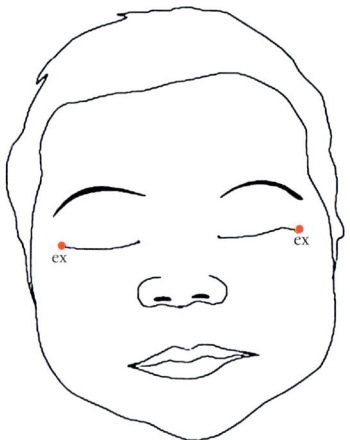

Figure 4

Fok TF, Hon KL, So HK, Wong E, Ng PC, Lee AK, Chang A. Craniofacial anthropometry of Hong Kong Chinese babies: the eye. Orthod Craniofac Res 2003;6:48–53.

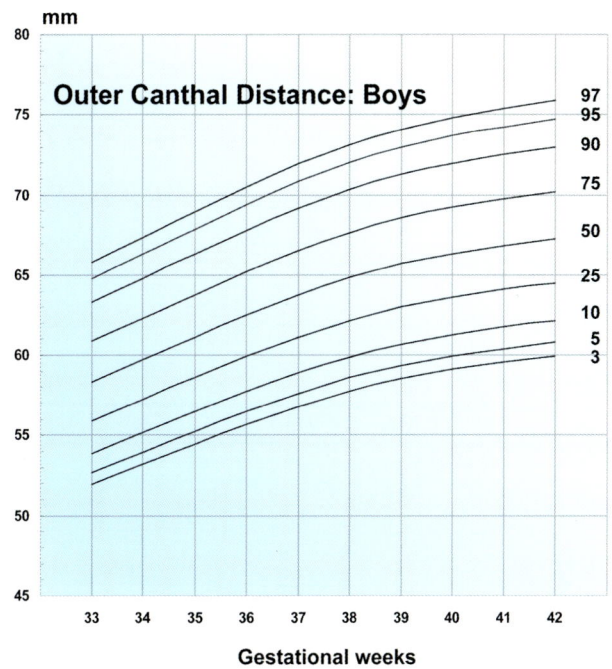

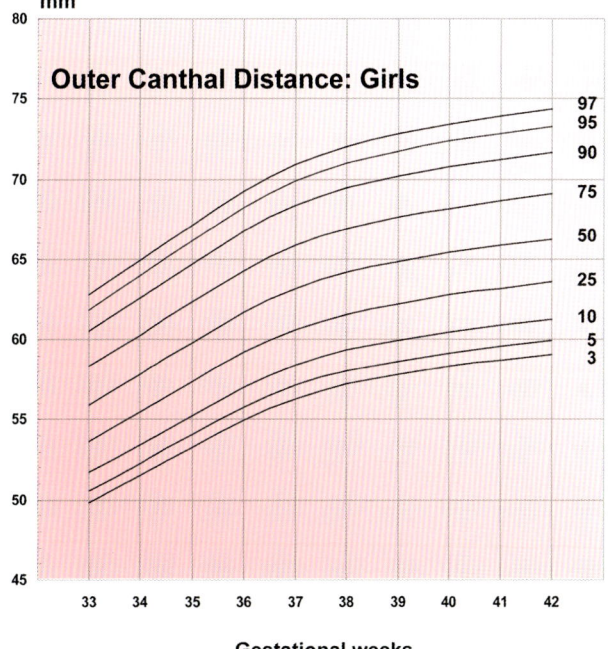

INNER CANTHAL DISTANCE

Definition	The distance between the inner canthi of the two eyes (en-en) in millimetres.
Instrument	Spreading caliper.
Remark	The distance from the innermost corner of one eye to the innermost corner of the other eye, in a straight line avoiding the curvature of the face.

Inner canthal distance (mm)

	Boys			Girls		
Gestation (wk)	N	Mean	SD	N	Mean	SD
33	10	17	2	5	17	2
34	9	17	2	11	17	2
35	16	17	1	15	17	2
36	37	18	2	28	17	2
37	125	18	2	112	18	2
38	241	18	2	234	18	2
39	358	18	2	279	18	2
40	294	19	2	268	18	2
41	138	19	2	120	18	2
42	40	19	2	37	18	2

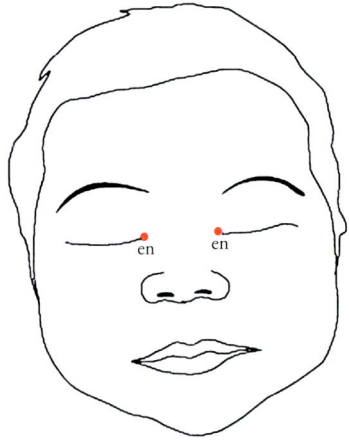

Figure 5

Fok TF, Hon KL, So HK, Wong E, Ng PC, Lee AK, Chang A. *Craniofacial anthropometry of Hong Kong Chinese babies: the eye. Orthod Craniofac Res 2003;6:48–53.*

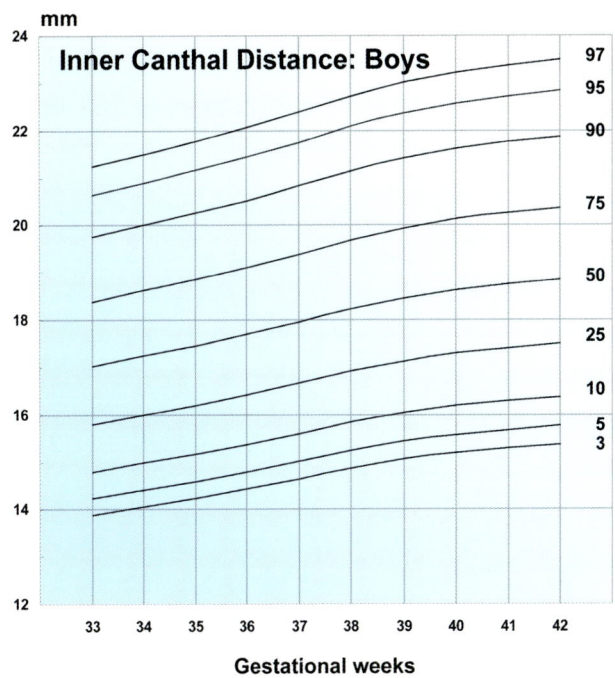

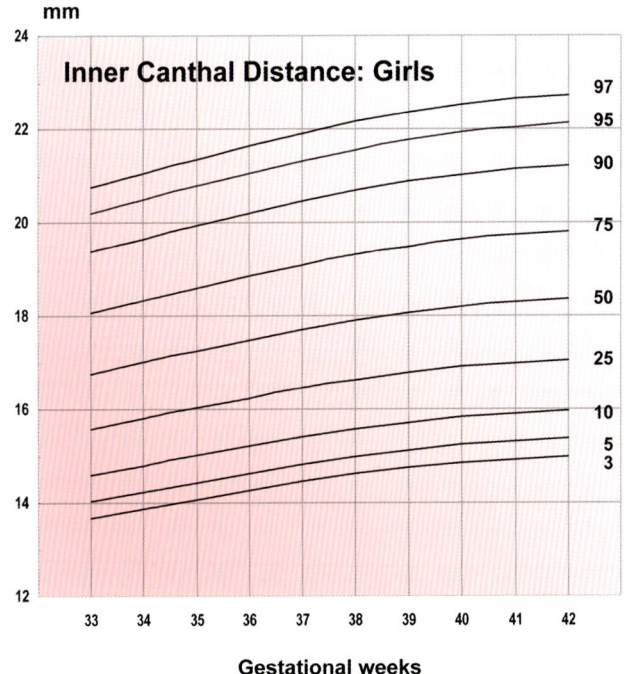

PALPEBRAL FISSURE LENGTH

Definition   The distance between the inner and outer canthus of one eye (en-ex) in millimetres.
Instrument   Spreading caliper.
Remark   Measure from the inner to the outer canthus of the eye.

Palpebral fissure length (mm)

Gestation (wk)	Boys			Girls		
	N	Mean	SD	N	Mean	SD
33	10	41	4	5	39	5
34	9	42	4	11	41	5
35	16	44	5	15	43	4
36	37	45	5	28	44	4
37	125	46	5	112	45	5
38	241	47	4	234	46	5
39	358	47	4	279	47	5
40	294	48	4	268	47	4
41	138	48	4	120	48	4
42	40	48	4	37	48	4

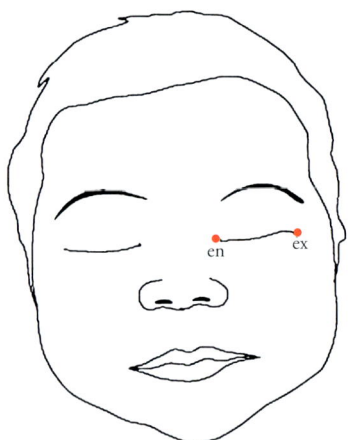

Figure 6

Fok TF, Hon KL, So HK, Wong E, Ng PC, Lee AK, Chang A. Craniofacial anthropometry of Hong Kong Chinese babies: the eye. Orthod Craniofac Res 2003;6:48–53.

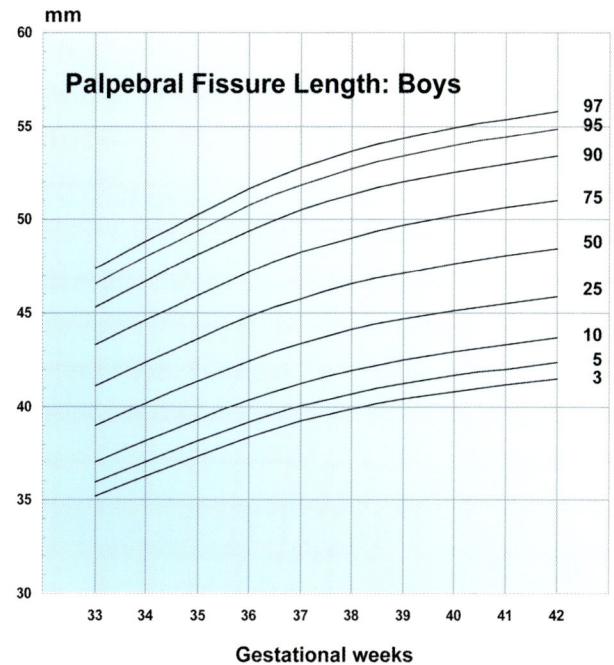

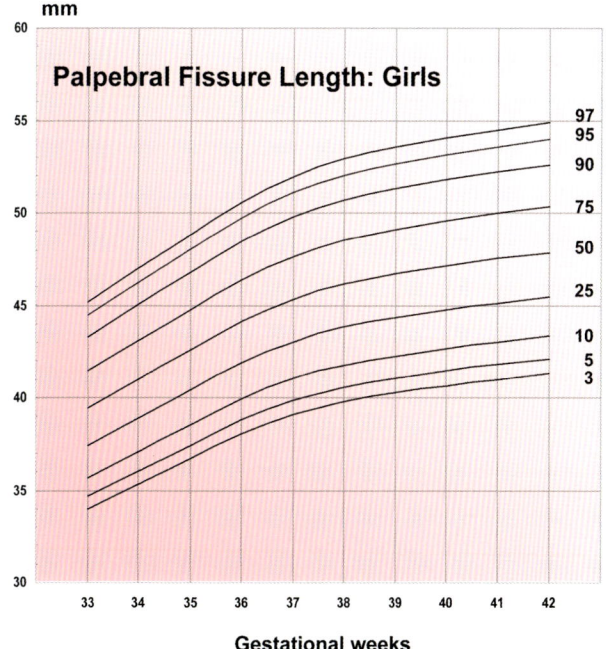

NASAL LENGTH

Definition	The distance from the nasal root to the nasal base (se-sn) in millimetres.
Instrument	Spreading caliper.
Remark	The distance from the deepest depression at the root of the nose to the deepest concavity at the base of the nose, in a vertical axis.

Nasal length (mm)

	Boys			Girls		
Gestation (wk)	N	Mean	SD	N	Mean	SD
33	10	17	1	5	16	1
34	9	17	2	11	16	2
35	16	17	1	15	17	2
36	37	17	1	28	17	2
37	125	17	2	112	17	2
38	241	18	2	234	17	2
39	358	18	2	279	17	2
40	294	18	2	268	17	2
41	138	18	2	120	17	2
42	40	18	2	37	17	2

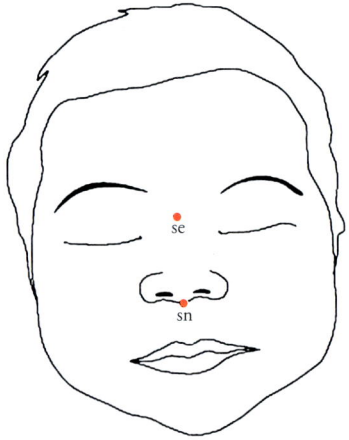

Figure 7

Fok TF, Hon KL, So HK, Wong E, Ng PC, Lee AK, Chang A. *Facial anthropometry of Hong Kong Chinese babies. Orthod Craniofac Res 2003;6:164–72.*

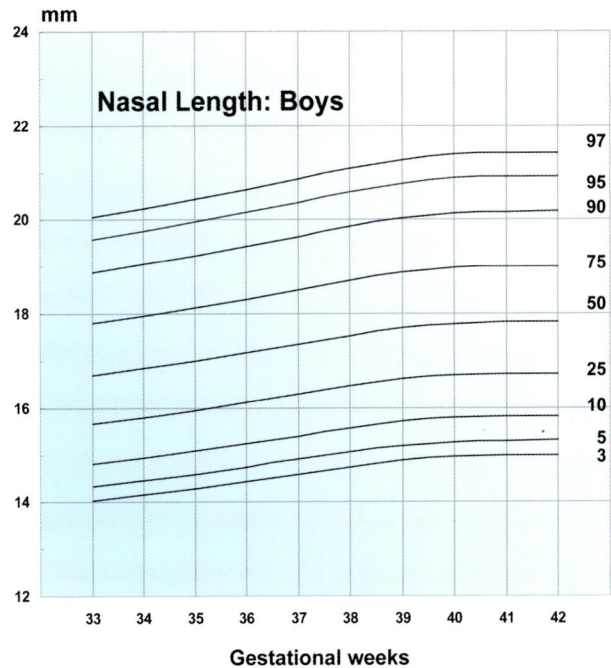

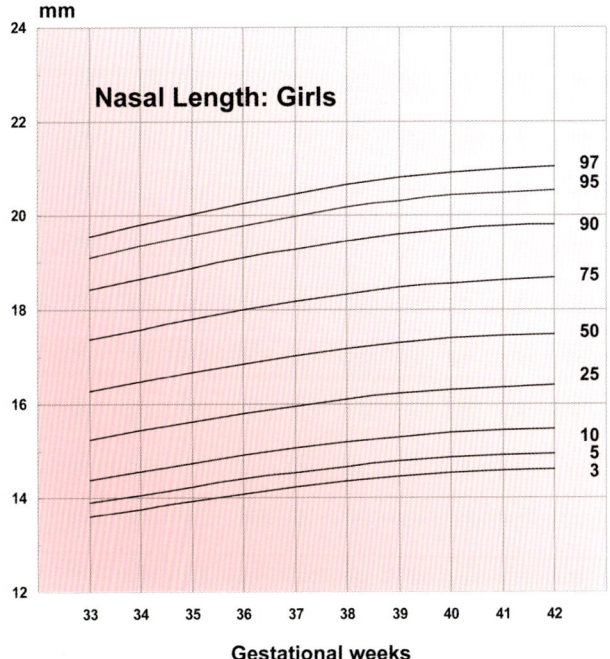

NASAL WIDTH (INTERALAR DISTANCE)

Definition   Distance between the most lateral aspect of one ala nasi to the lateral-most aspect of the other ala nasi (al-al) in millimetres.

Instrument   Spreading caliper.

Remark   The distance from the lateral-most aspect of one ala nasi to the lateral-most aspect of the other ala nasi.

Nasal width (mm)

Gestation (wk)	Boys			Girls		
	N	Mean	SD	N	Mean	SD
33	10	19	2	5	19	2
34	9	20	2	11	20	2
35	16	20	2	15	20	1
36	37	21	1	28	20	2
37	125	21	2	112	21	2
38	241	21	2	234	21	2
39	358	22	2	279	21	2
40	294	22	2	268	21	2
41	138	22	2	120	21	2
42	40	22	2	37	21	2

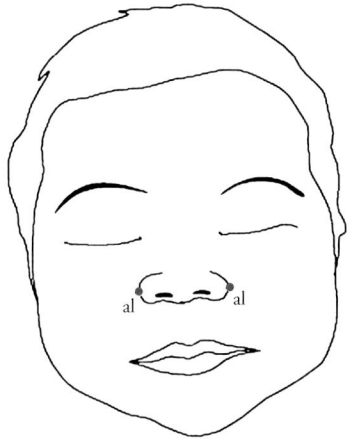

Figure 8

Fok TF, Hon KL, So HK, Wong E, Ng PC, Lee AK, Chang A. Facial anthropometry of Hong Kong Chinese babies. Orthod Craniofac Res 2003;6:164–72.

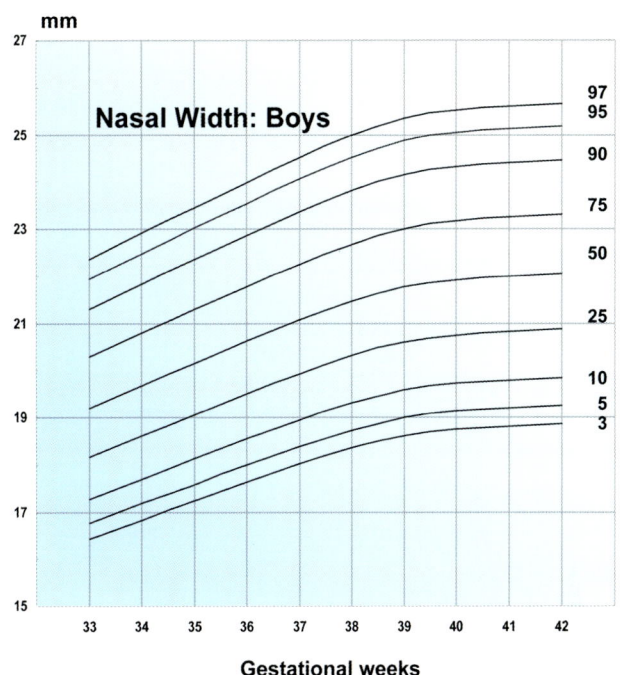

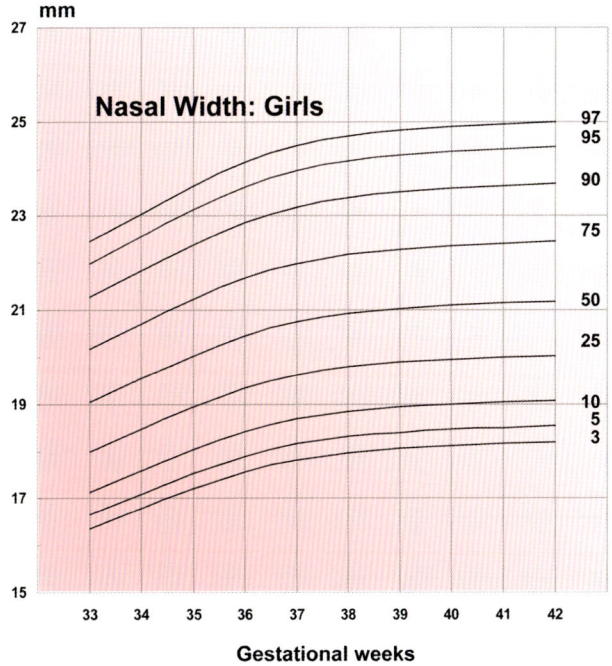

EAR LENGTH

Definition   Maximum distance from the superior aspect to the inferior aspect of the external ear in millimetres.

Instrument   Spreading caliper.

Remark   The distance from the superior aspect of the outer rim of the helix to the most inferior border of the earlobe.

Ear length (mm)

Gestation (wk)	Boys			Girls		
	N	Mean	SD	N	Mean	SD
33	10	30	4	5	30	3
34	9	30	2	11	30	2
35	16	31	3	15	30	3
36	37	31	3	28	31	3
37	125	32	3	112	31	3
38	241	32	3	234	31	3
39	358	32	3	279	31	3
40	294	32	3	268	32	3
41	138	33	3	120	32	3
42	40	33	3	37	32	3

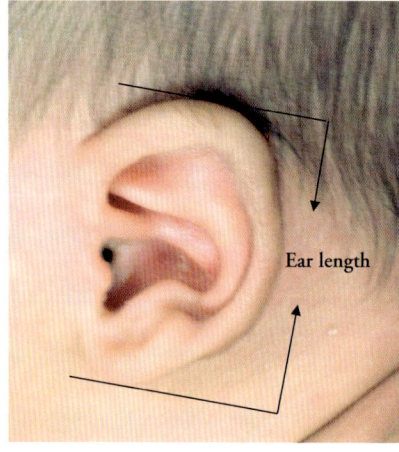

Figure 9

Fok TF, Hon KL, So HK, Ng PC, Wong E, Lee AK, Chang A. Auricular anthropometry of Hong Kong Chinese babies. Orthod Craniofac Res 2004;7:10–4.

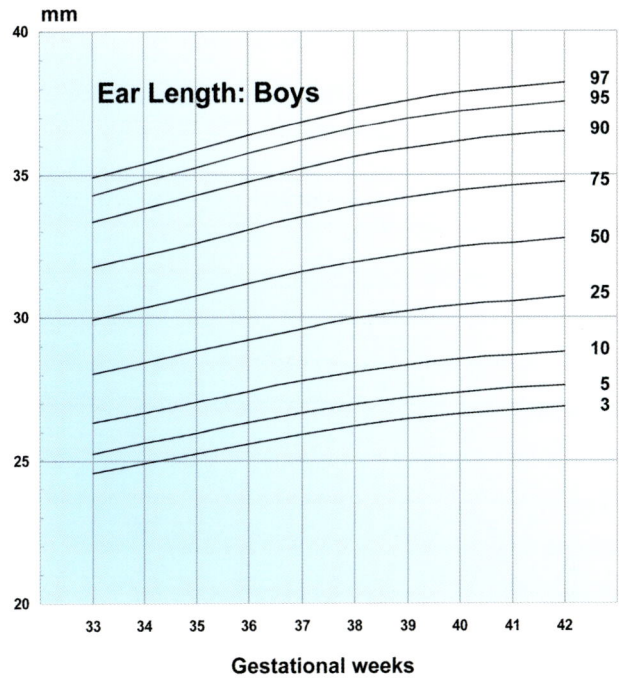

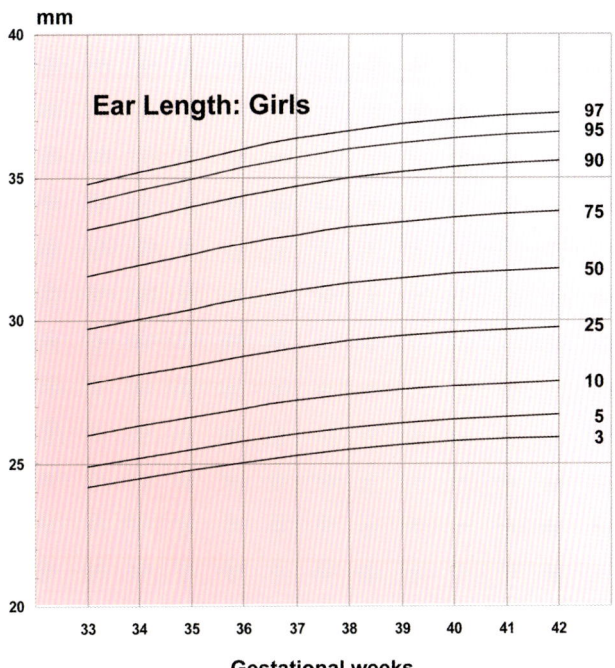

EAR WIDTH

Definition	Width of external ears (pinna) in millimetres.
Instrument	Spreading caliper.
Remark	The distance transverses from the anterior base of the tragus, which can be palpated, through the region of the external auditory canal to the margin of the helical rim, at the widest point.

Ear width (mm)

	Boys			Girls		
Gestation (wk)	N	Mean	SD	N	Mean	SD
33	10	21	3	5	19	2
34	9	21	2	11	20	2
35	16	22	2	15	20	2
36	37	22	2	28	21	2
37	125	22	2	112	22	2
38	241	23	2	234	22	2
39	358	23	2	279	22	2
40	294	23	2	268	22	2
41	138	23	2	120	22	2
42	40	24	2	37	22	2

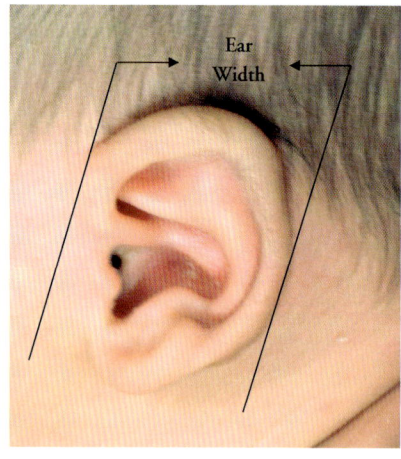

Figure 10

Fok TF, Hon KL, So HK, Ng PC, Wong E, Lee AK, Chang A. Auricular anthropometry of Hong Kong Chinese babies. Orthod Craniofac Res 2004;7:10–4.

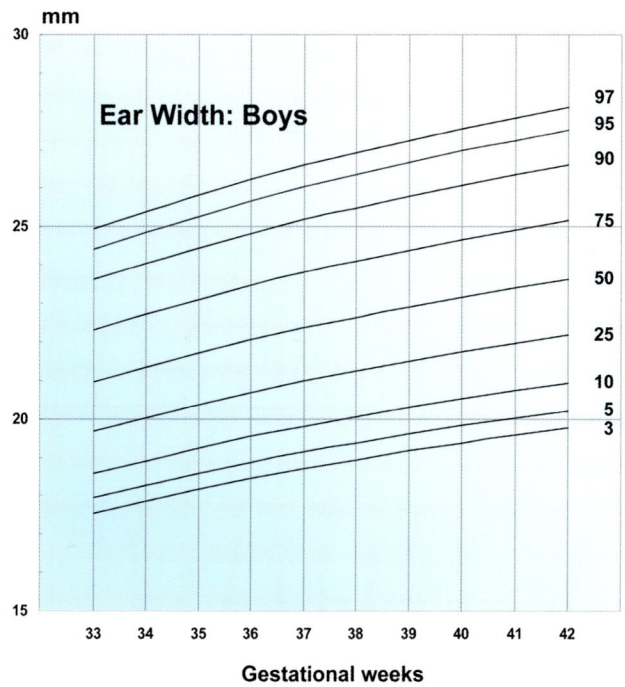

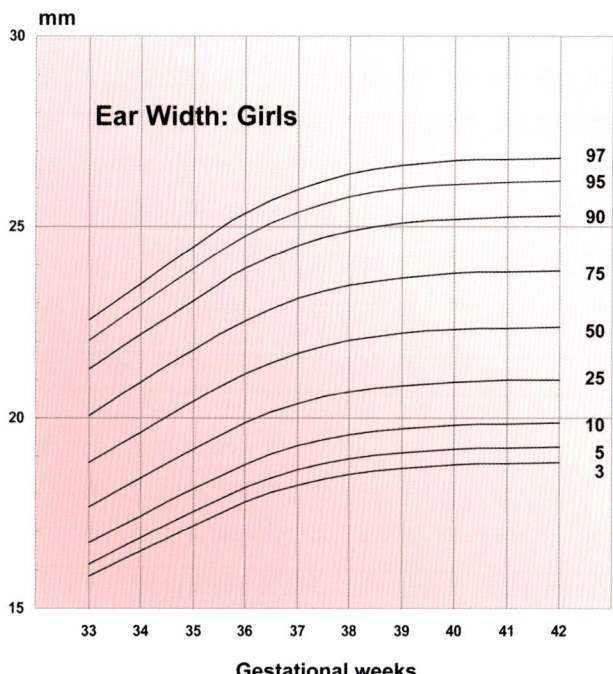

PHILTRUM LENGTH

Definition	Distance between the base of the nose and the border of the upper lip, in the midline (sn-ls) in millimetres.
Instrument	A straight-edged ruler.
Remark	The distance from the base of the nose to the superior aspect of the vermilion border of the lip, in the midline.

Philtrum length (mm)

	Boys			Girls		
Gestation (wk)	N	Mean	SD	N	Mean	SD
33	10	8	1	5	8	1
34	9	8	1	11	8	1
35	16	8	1	15	8	1
36	37	9	1	28	8	1
37	125	9	1	112	9	1
38	241	9	1	234	9	1
39	358	9	1	279	9	1
40	294	9	1	268	9	1
41	138	9	1	120	9	1
42	40	9	1	37	9	1

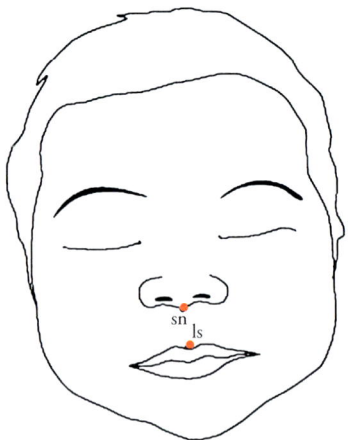

Figure 11

Fok TF, Hon KL, So HK, Wong E, Ng PC, Lee AK, Chang A. *Facial anthropometry of Hong Kong Chinese babies. Orthod Craniofac Res 2003;6:164–72.*

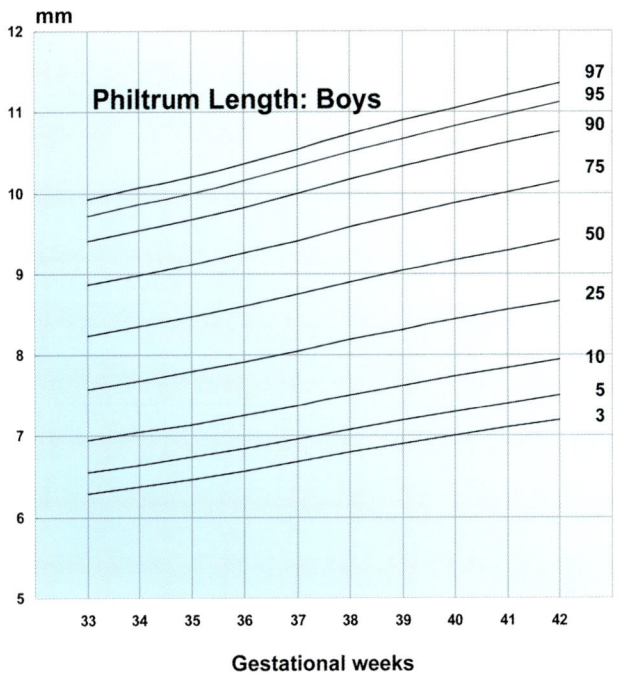

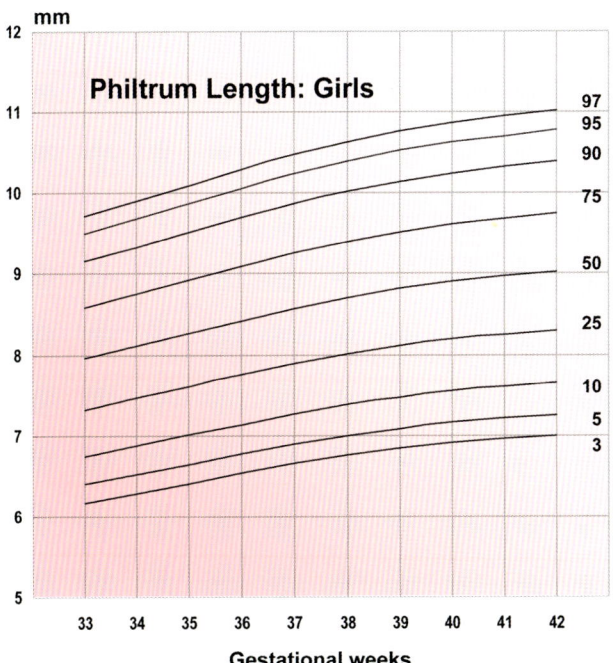

LIMBS

- Arm Length
- Arm Circumference
- Upper Arm Length
- Lower Arm Length
- Leg Length
- Thigh Circumference
- Upper Leg Length
- Lower Leg Length

ARM LENGTH (Total Upper Limb Length)

Definition   Length of the whole arm (the arm and hand combined) in millimetres.

Instrument   Inelastic tape measure.

Remark   The distance between the acromion and the tip of the middle finger.

Arm length (mm)

Gestation (wk)	Boys			Girls		
	N	Mean	SD	N	Mean	SD
28	27	158	11	19	152	11
29	26	165	13	36	159	11
30	51	172	11	24	167	13
31	41	179	16	25	174	17
32	36	185	16	45	181	15
33	89	191	15	65	187	14
34	101	197	13	110	193	13
35	148	202	14	133	198	15
36	275	206	10	211	203	11
37	432	210	12	351	207	12
38	1054	214	11	872	211	11
39	1304	217	11	1218	214	11
40	1179	220	11	1098	216	11
41	544	222	12	505	219	12
42	115	225	12	92	221	12

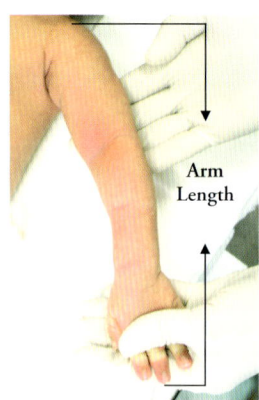

Figure 12

Fok TF, Hon KL, Ng PC, Wong E, So HK, Lau J, Chow CB, Lee WH; Hong Kong Neonatal Measurements Working Group. Limbs anthropometry of singleton Chinese newborns of 28–42 weeks' gestation. Biol Neonate 2006;89:25–34.

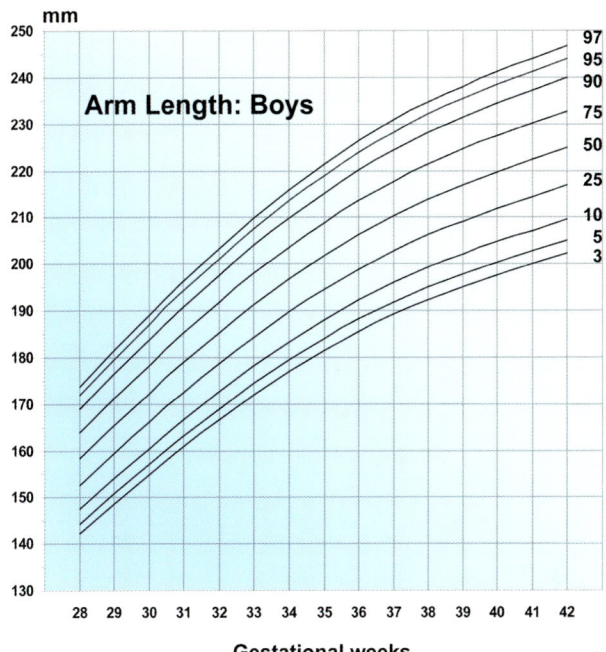

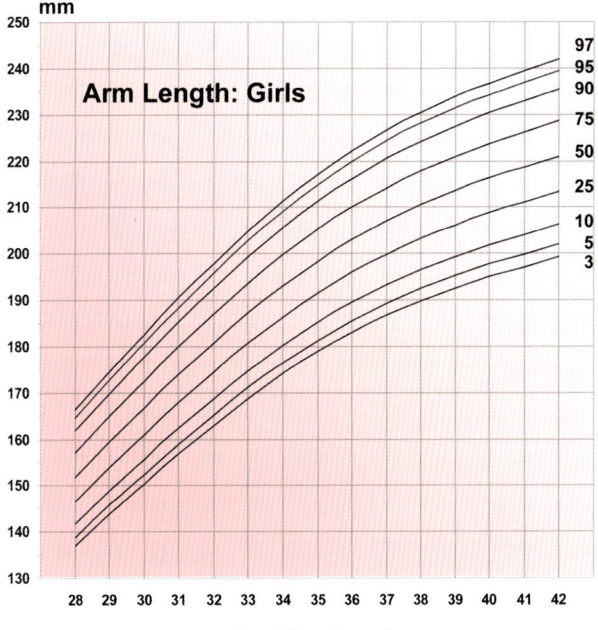

ARM CIRCUMFERENCE

Definition	Maximum circumference of the arm in millimetres.
Instrument	Inelastic tape measure.
Remark	Measurement is taken at the widest point at the biceps, just below the insertion of the deltoid.

Arm circumference (mm)

	Boys			Girls		
Gestation (wk)	N	Mean	SD	N	Mean	SD
28	27	65	15	19	65	5
29	26	69	10	36	69	7
30	51	73	4	24	72	9
31	41	77	11	25	76	11
32	36	81	11	45	80	9
33	89	85	10	65	83	8
34	101	88	8	110	87	10
35	148	91	8	133	91	12
36	275	95	8	211	94	8
37	432	98	8	351	97	9
38	1054	100	8	872	99	8
39	1304	102	8	1218	101	8
40	1179	104	8	1098	103	8
41	544	106	9	505	105	8
42	115	108	7	92	107	8

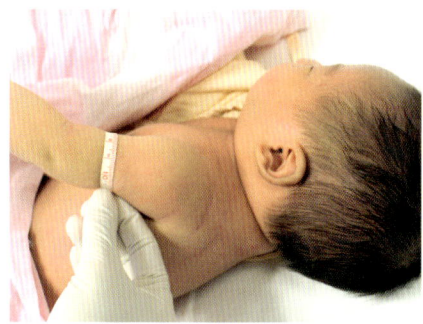

Figure 13

Fok TF, Hon KL, Ng PC, Wong E, So HK, Lau J, Chow CB, Lee WH; Hong Kong Neonatal Measurements Working Group. Limbs anthropometry of singleton Chinese newborns of 28–42 weeks' gestation. Biol Neonate 2006;89:25–34.

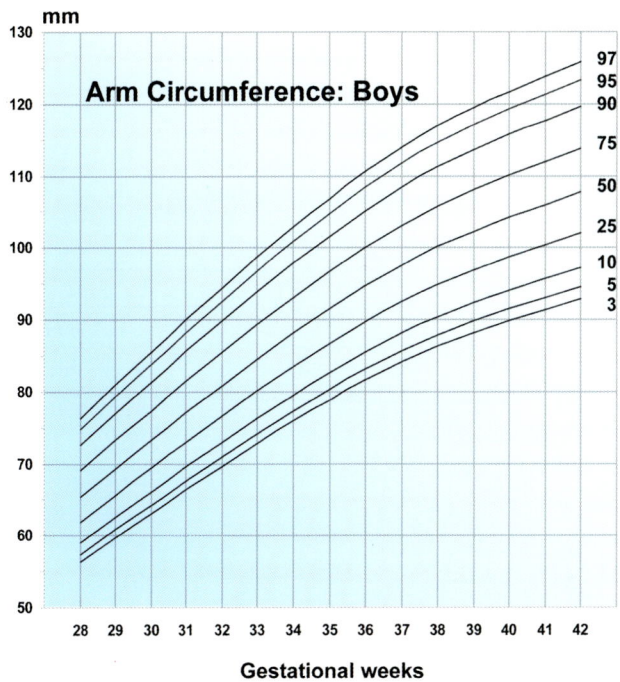

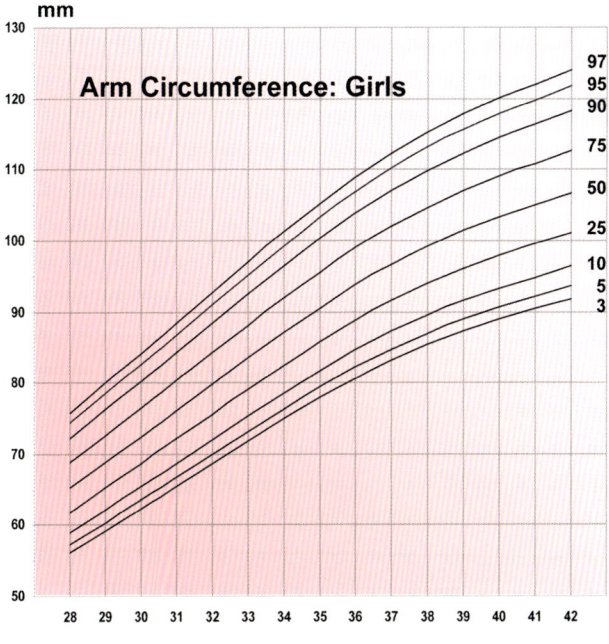

UPPER ARM LENGTH

Definition   Length of the upper arm in millimetres.
Instrument   Spreading caliper.
Remark   The distance from the acromion along the posterior lateral aspect of
the arm to the distal medial border of the olecranon.

Upper arm length (mm)

Gestation (wk)	Boys			Girls		
	N	Mean	SD	N	Mean	SD
28	27	72	6	19	69	6
29	26	75	4	36	73	5
30	51	78	5	24	76	5
31	41	81	5	25	80	7
32	36	84	9	45	83	7
33	89	87	8	65	86	7
34	101	89	7	110	88	8
35	148	91	7	133	90	7
36	275	93	5	211	92	5
37	432	95	5	351	94	6
38	1054	97	5	872	95	5
39	1304	98	5	1218	96	5
40	1179	99	5	1098	97	5
41	544	100	5	505	98	6
42	115	101	5	92	99	6

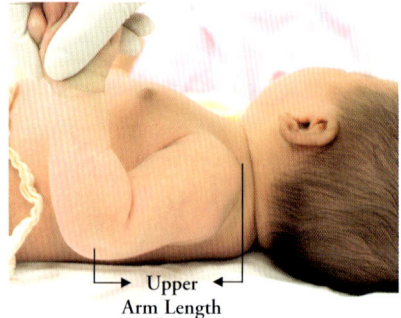

Upper
Arm Length

Figure 14

Fok TF, Hon KL, Ng PC, Wong E, So HK, Lau J, Chow CB, Lee WH; Hong Kong Neonatal Measurements Working Group. Limbs anthropometry of singleton Chinese newborns of 28–42 weeks' gestation. Biol Neonate 2006;89:25–34.

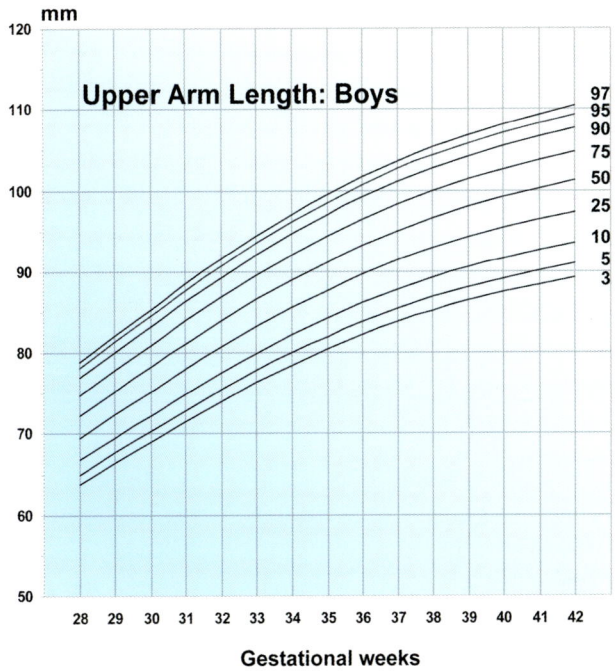

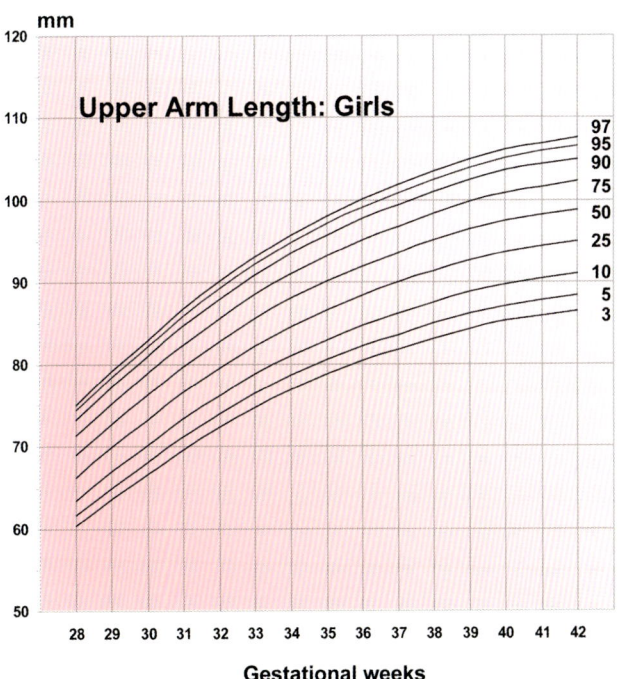

LOWER ARM LENGTH (FOREARM LENGTH)

Definition   Length of the forearm in millimetres.
Instrument   Spreading caliper.
Remark   The distance from the most prominent point of the olecranon to the distal lateral process of the radius along the lateral surface of the forearm.

Lower arm length (mm)

Gestation (wk)	Boys			Girls		
	N	Mean	SD	N	Mean	SD
28	27	61	4	19	59	2
29	26	63	3	36	61	3
30	51	65	4	24	63	3
31	41	67	5	25	65	7
32	36	69	6	45	67	6
33	89	71	6	65	69	4
34	101	72	5	110	71	6
35	148	74	5	133	72	6
36	275	75	4	211	74	4
37	432	77	5	351	75	5
38	1054	78	4	872	76	4
39	1304	79	4	1218	78	4
40	1179	80	5	1098	78	5
41	544	81	5	505	79	5
42	115	82	5	92	80	5

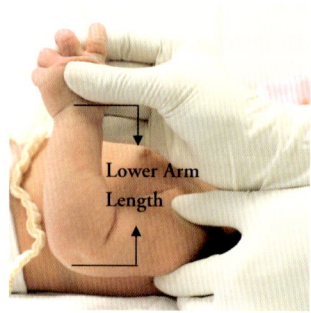

Figure 15

Fok TF, Hon KL, Ng PC, Wong E, So HK, Lau J, Chow CB, Lee WH; Hong Kong Neonatal Measurements Working Group. Limbs anthropometry of singleton Chinese newborns of 28–42 weeks' gestation. Biol Neonate 2006;89:25–34.

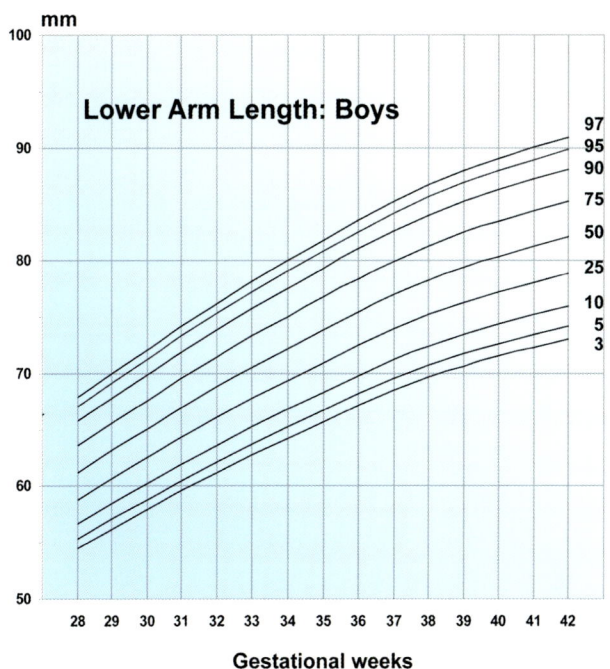

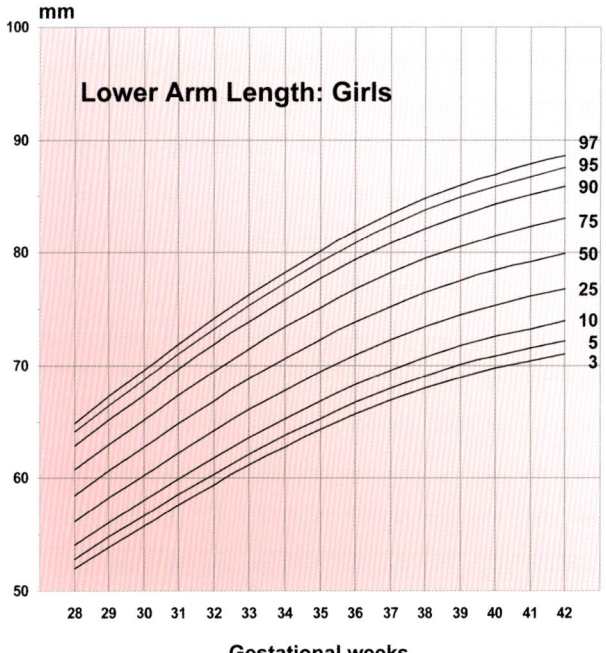

LEG LENGTH

Definition   The sum of the length of the upper leg length and the lower leg length in millimetres.

Instrument   Inelastic tape measure.

Remark   Leg length is measured from the greater trochanter of the femur to the lateral malleolus of the ankle along the lateral aspect of the leg with the baby lying supine.

Leg length (mm)

Gestation (wk)	Boys			Girls		
	N	Mean	SD	N	Mean	SD
28	27	137	11	19	138	12
29	26	144	18	36	144	14
30	51	150	10	24	150	12
31	41	156	16	25	155	16
32	36	162	13	45	161	13
33	89	168	13	65	166	12
34	101	173	13	110	172	13
35	148	178	10	133	176	12
36	275	182	9	211	180	9
37	432	186	10	351	184	10
38	1054	189	9	872	187	9
39	1304	192	9	1218	190	9
40	1179	195	10	1098	192	10
41	544	197	10	505	194	10
42	115	200	11	92	196	11

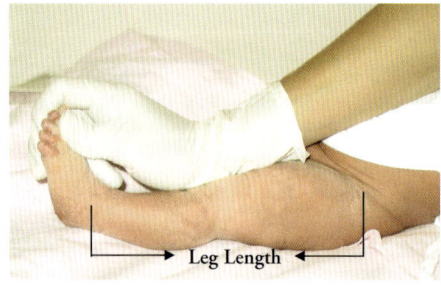

Figure 16

Fok TF, Hon KL, Ng PC, Wong E, So HK, Lau J, Chow CB, Lee WH; Hong Kong Neonatal Measurements Working Group. Limbs anthropometry of singleton Chinese newborns of 28–42 weeks' gestation. Biol Neonate 2006;89:25–34.

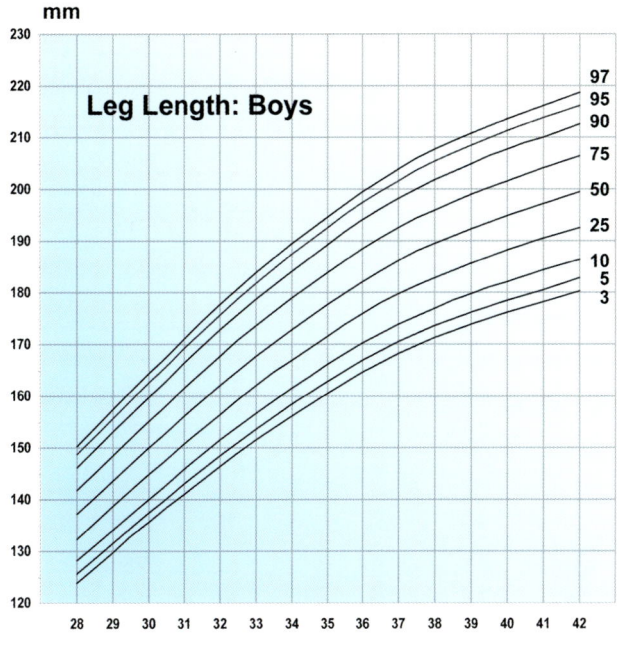

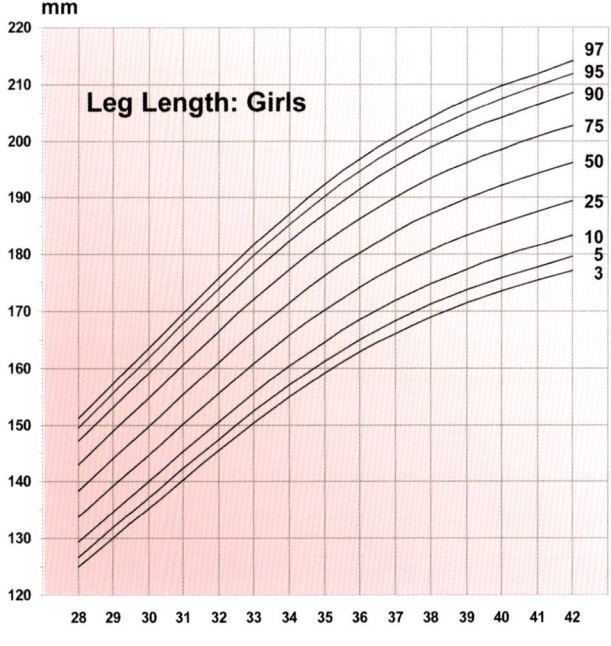

THIGH CIRCUMFERENCE

Definition	Maximum circumference of the upper leg in millimetres.
Instrument	Inelastic tape measure.
Remark	The widest circumference just below the gluteal crease.

Thigh circumference (mm)

Gestation (wk)	Boys			Girls		
	N	Mean	SD	N	Mean	SD
28	27	96	15	19	93	12
29	26	101	11	36	98	11
30	51	106	5	24	103	10
31	41	112	14	25	109	16
32	36	118	18	45	115	16
33	89	124	16	65	122	16
34	101	130	13	110	130	14
35	148	137	14	133	137	16
36	275	143	14	211	143	13
37	432	148	13	351	148	13
38	1054	152	13	872	152	13
39	1304	155	12	1218	155	12
40	1179	158	13	1098	157	13
41	544	160	13	505	159	12
42	115	162	14	92	160	13

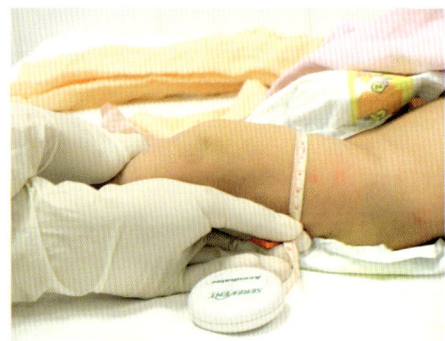

Figure 17

Fok TF, Hon KL, Ng PC, Wong E, So HK, Lau J, Chow CB, Lee WH; Hong Kong Neonatal Measurements Working Group. Limbs anthropometry of singleton Chinese newborns of 28–42 weeks' gestation. Biol Neonate 2006;89:25–34.

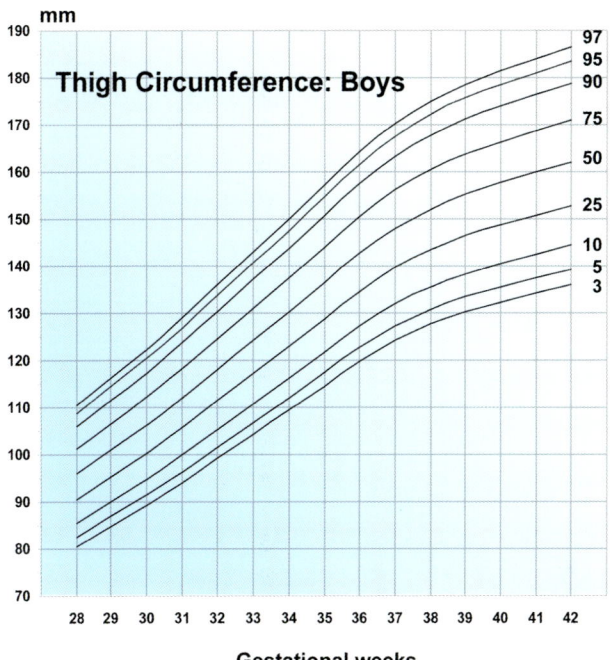

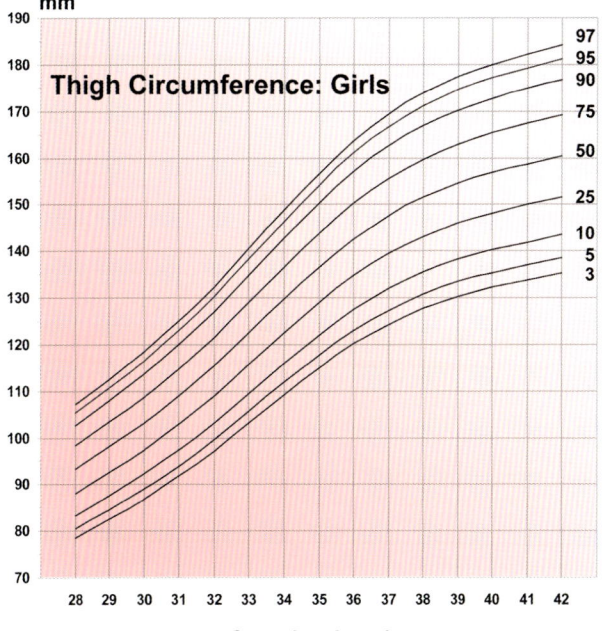

UPPER LEG LENGTH

Definition   Length of the upper leg in millimetres.
Instrument   Spreading caliper.
Remark   The distance from the greater trochanter of the femur to the
              proximal lateral tibial condyle along the lateral aspect of the leg.

Upper leg length (mm)

Gestation (wk)	Boys			Girls		
	N	Mean	SD	N	Mean	SD
28	27	75	5	19	76	9
29	26	78	4	36	79	8
30	51	82	7	24	82	4
31	41	85	9	25	85	7
32	36	88	7	45	88	6
33	89	91	8	65	91	8
34	101	94	9	110	93	7
35	148	96	6	133	96	8
36	275	99	6	211	98	5
37	432	101	5	351	100	6
38	1054	102	5	872	101	5
39	1304	104	5	1218	103	5
40	1179	105	5	1098	104	5
41	544	106	6	505	105	5
42	115	108	6	92	106	7

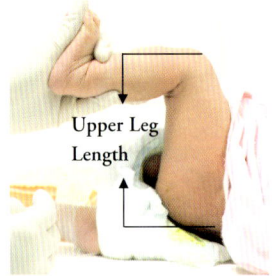

Figure 18

Fok TF, Hon KL, Ng PC, Wong E, So HK, Lau J, Chow CB, Lee WH; Hong Kong Neonatal Measurements Working Group. Limbs anthropometry of singleton Chinese newborns of 28–42 weeks' gestation. Biol Neonate 2006;89:25–34.

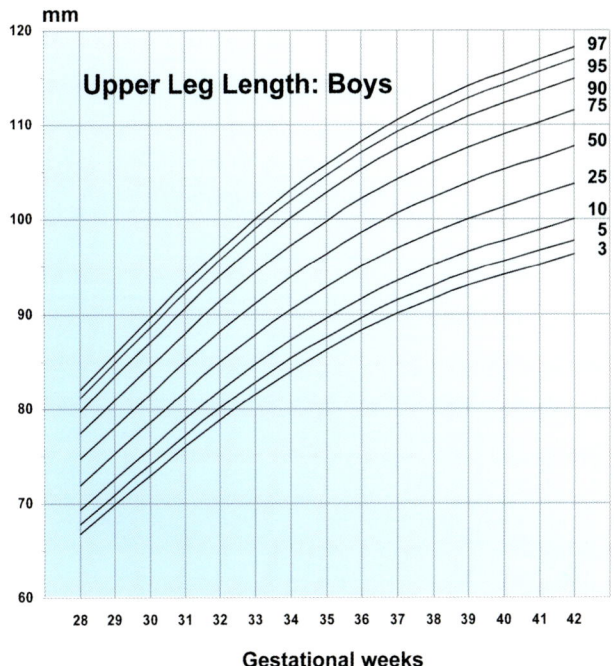

Gestational weeks

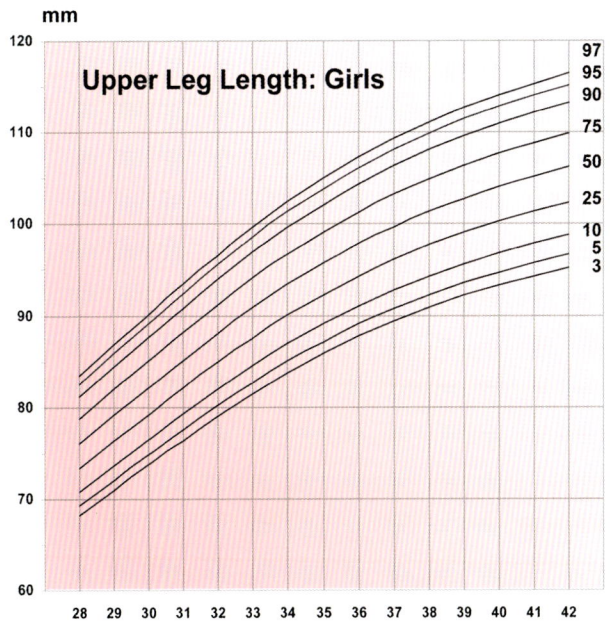

Gestational weeks

LOWER LEG LENGTH

Definition	Length of the lower leg in millimetres.
Instrument	Spreading caliper.
Remark	The distance from the lateral upper condyle of the tibia to the lateral malleolus of the ankle.

Lower leg length (mm)

Gestation (wk)	Boys			Girls		
	N	Mean	SD	N	Mean	SD
28	27	64	6	19	64	6
29	26	67	2	36	67	3
30	51	70	6	24	69	5
31	41	72	9	25	72	8
32	36	75	5	45	74	6
33	89	77	5	65	77	6
34	101	79	5	110	79	6
35	148	82	6	133	81	6
36	275	84	5	211	82	5
37	432	85	5	351	84	5
38	1054	87	5	872	85	5
39	1304	88	5	1218	87	5
40	1179	90	5	1098	88	5
41	544	91	6	505	89	5
42	115	92	6	92	89	6

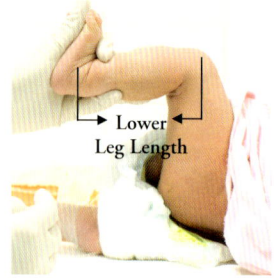

Figure 19

Fok TF, Hon KL, Ng PC, Wong E, So HK, Lau J, Chow CB, Lee WH; Hong Kong Neonatal Measurements Working Group. Limbs anthropometry of singleton Chinese newborns of 28–42 weeks' gestation. Biol Neonate 2006;89:25–34.

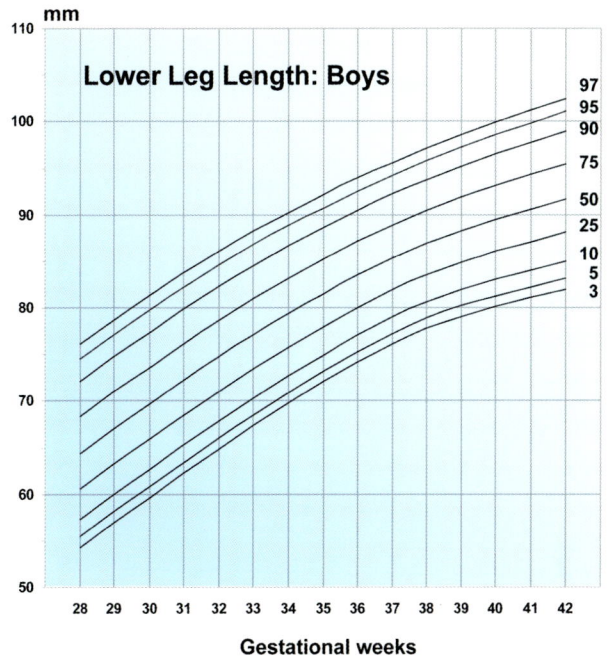

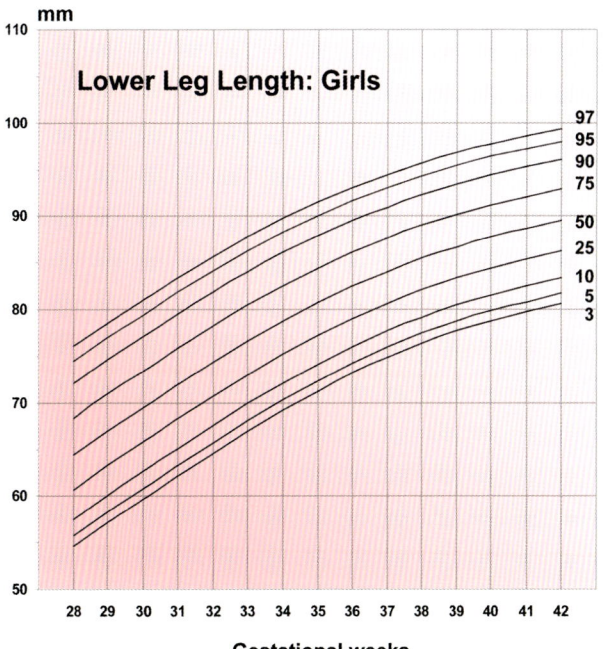

GENITALIA

PENILE LENGTH

Definition   The length of the gently stretched penis from the base to the tip in millimetres.

Instrument   A straight-edged ruler.

Remark   The distance from the base of the penis (pubic ramus) to the tip of the glans with the penis gently stretched. The glans of the penis may need to be palpated through the foreskin in individuals who are not circumcised.

Penile Length (mm)

Gestation (wk)	N	Mean	SD
37	383	29	4
38	908	30	4
39	1151	30	4
40	1026	30	4
41	469	31	5
42	100	31	5

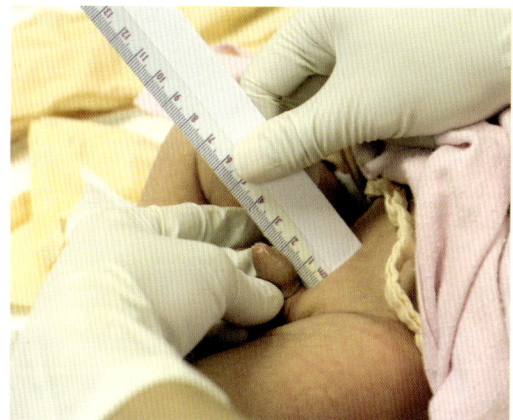

Figure 20

Fok TF, Hon KL, So HK, Wong E, Ng PC, Chang A, Lau J, Chow CB, Lee WH; Hong Kong Neonatal Measurements Working Group. Normative data of penile length for term Chinese newborns. Biol Neonate 2005;87:242–5.

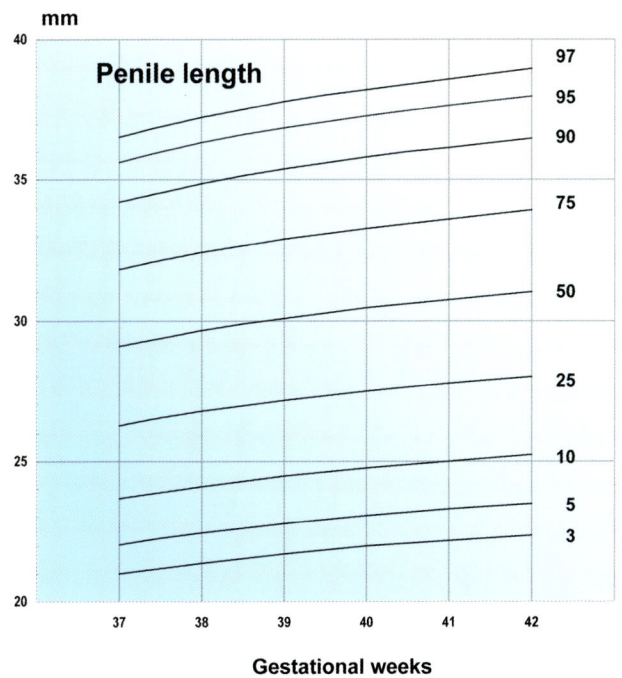

Gestational weeks

SKINFOLD THICKNESS

- **Triceps Skinfold Thickness**
- **Subscapular Skinfold Thickness**

Method   A skinfold (subcutaneous fold without muscle) was held between the investigator's thumb and index finger. The caliper was placed about 1 mm below the left hand, perpendicular to the skinfold. The caliper was held in the right hand and the measurement was read within 3 seconds (so as to avoid prolonged compression of the subcutaneous tissue).

TRICEPS SKINFOLD THICKNESS

Definition	Skinfold thickness of triceps in millimetres.
Instrument	Skinfold caliper.
Remark	Triceps skinfold is measured over the mid-point of the muscle belly, mid-way between the olecranon and the tip of the acromion, with the left upper arm lying vertically. The reading is recorded within a few seconds once the dial comes to a halt, to the nearest 0.1mm.

Triceps skinfold (mm)

	Boys			Girls		
Gestation (wk)	N	Mean	SD	N	Mean	SD
31	41	3	1	25	3	1
32	36	3	1	45	4	1
33	89	4	1	65	4	1
34	101	4	1	110	4	1
35	148	4	1	133	4	1
36	275	4	1	211	4	1
37	432	4	1	351	4	1
38	1054	4	1	872	4	1
39	1304	4	1	1218	4	1
40	1179	5	1	1098	5	1
41	544	5	1	505	5	1
42	115	5	1	92	5	1

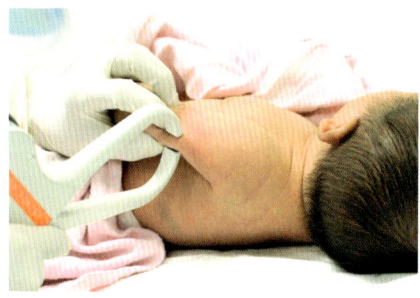

Figure 21

Fok TF, Hon KL, Wong E, Ng PC, So HK, Lau J, Chow CB, Lee WH; Hong Kong Neonatal Measurements Working Group. Normative data for triceps and subscapular skinfold thickness of Chinese Infants. Acta Paediatr 2006;95(12):161–9.

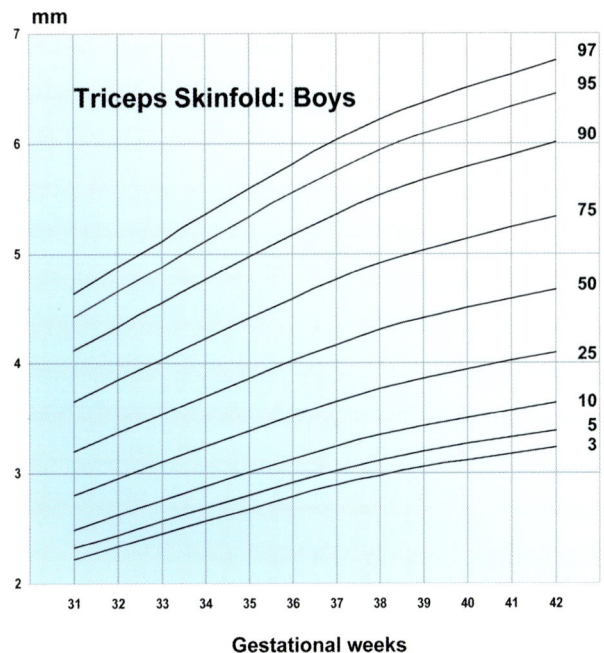

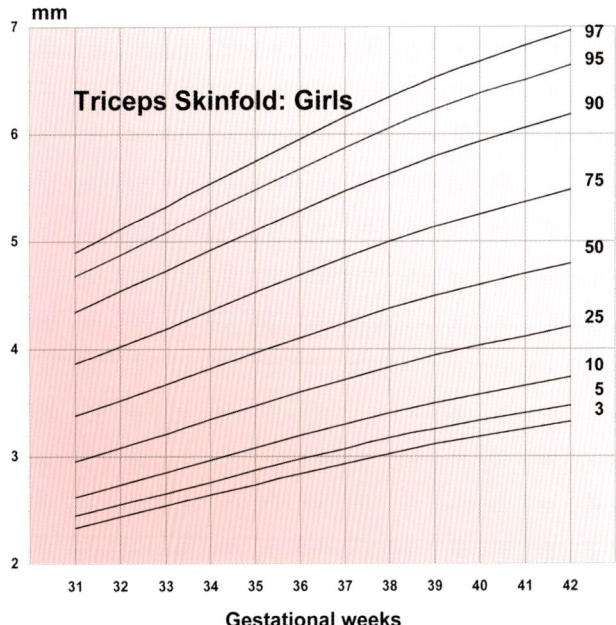

SUBSCAPULAR SKINFOLD THICKNESS

Definition	Skinfold thickness of the inferior angle of scapula in millimetres.
Instrument	Skinfold caliper.
	The caliper is designed to exert a constant pressure of $10g/mm^2$ at the opening and allow accuracy up to 0.1mm.
Remark	The Subscapular skinfold is measured immediately below the inferior angle of the left scapula.

Subscapular skinfold (mm)

	Boys			Girls		
Gestation (wk)	N	Mean	SD	N	Mean	SD
31	41	3	1	25	4	1
32	36	4	1	45	4	1
33	89	4	1	65	4	1
34	101	4	1	110	4	1
35	148	4	1	133	4	1
36	275	4	1	211	4	1
37	432	4	1	351	5	1
38	1054	5	1	872	5	1
39	1304	5	1	1218	5	1
40	1179	5	1	1098	5	1
41	544	5	1	505	5	1
42	115	5	1	92	5	1

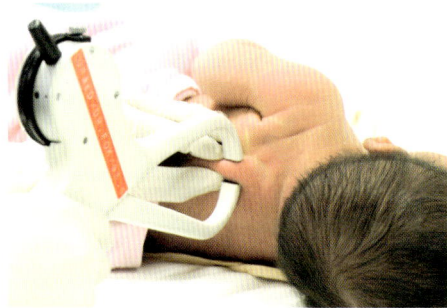

Figure 22

Fok TF, Hon KL, Wong E, Ng PC, So HK, Lau J, Chow CB, Lee WH; Hong Kong Neonatal Measurements Working Group. Normative data for triceps and subscapular skinfold thickness of Chinese Infants. Acta Paediatr 2006;95(12):161–9.

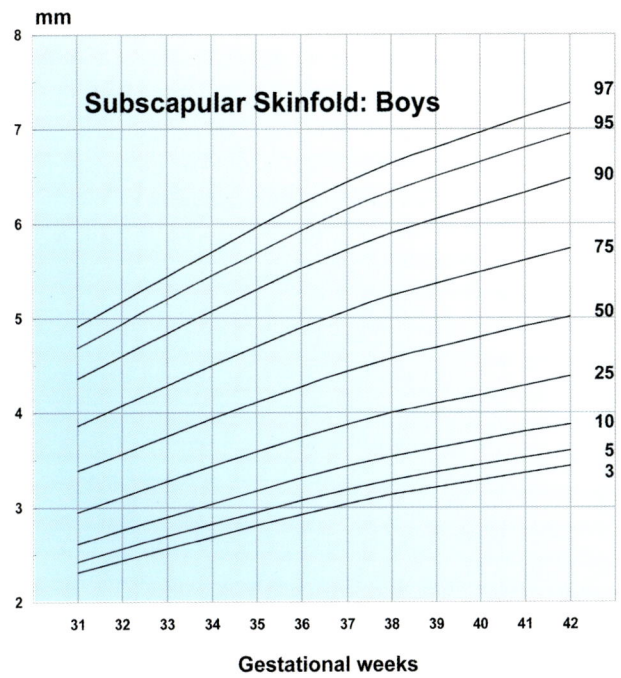

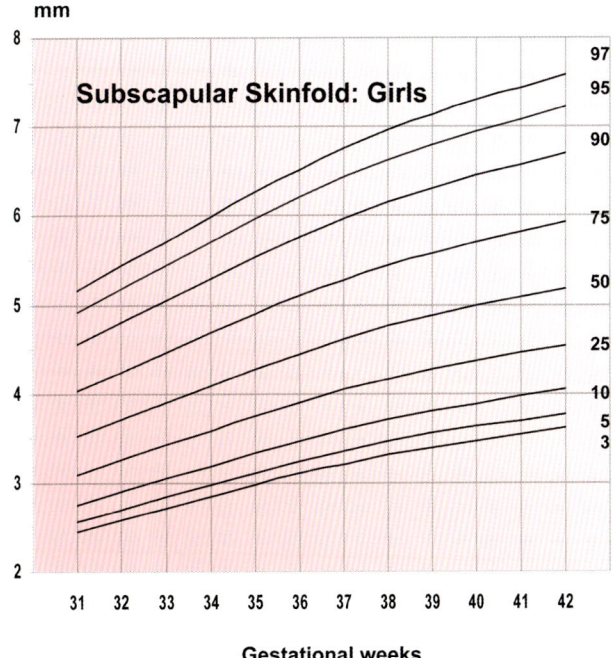

REFERENCES

Fok TF, So HK, Wong E, Ng PC, Chang A, Lau J, Chow CB, Lee WH; Hong Kong Neonatal Measurements Working Group. Updated gestational age specific birth weight, crown-heel length, and head circumference of Chinese newborns. Arch Dis Child Fetal Neonatal Ed 2003;88:F229–36.

Fok TF, Hon KL, So HK, Wong E, Ng PC, Lee AK, Chang A. Craniofacial anthropometry of Hong Kong Chinese babies: the eye. Orthod Craniofac Res 2003;6:48–53.

Fok TF, Hon KL, So HK, Wong E, Ng PC, Lee AK, Chang A. Facial anthropometry of Hong Kong Chinese babies. Orthod Craniofac Res 2003;6: 164–72.

Fok TF, Hon KL, So HK, Ng PC, Wong E, Lee AK, Chang A. Auricular anthropometry of Hong Kong Chinese babies. Orthod Craniofac Res 2004;7: 10–4.

Fok TF, Hon KL, So HK, Wong E, Ng PC, Chang A, Lau J, Chow CB, Lee WH; Hong Kong Neonatal Measurements Working Group. Normative data of penile length for term Chinese newborns. Biol Neonate 2005;87:242–5.

Fok TF, Hon KL, Wong E, Ng PC, So HK, Lau J, Chow CB, Lee WH; Hong Kong Neonatal Measurements Working Group. Trunk anthropometry of Hong Kong Chinese infants. Early Hum Dev 2005;81:781–90.

Fok TF, Hon KL, Ng PC, Wong E, So HK, Lau J, Chow CB, Lee WH; Hong Kong Neonatal Measurements Working Group. Limbs anthropometry of singleton Chinese newborns of 28–42 weeks' gestation. Biol Neonate 2006;89: 25–34.

Fok TF, Hon KL, Ng PC, Wong E, So HK, Lau TF, Chow CB, Lee WH; Hong Kong Neonatal Measurements Working Group. Normative data for triceps and subscapular skinfold thickness of Chinese Infants. Acta Paediatr 2006;95(12): 161–9.

Hall JG, Froster-Iskenius UG, Allanson JE. Handbook of Normal Physical Measurements. 1989. New York: Oxford University Press.